Rx for the Nursing Shortage

A GUIDEBOOK

Rx for the Nursing Shortage

A G U I D E B O O K

Julie W. Schaffner and Patti Ludwig-Beymer

ACHE Management Series

Health Administration Press

The American Organization of Nurse Executives

Your board, staff, or clients may also benefit from this book's insight. For more information on quantity discounts, contact the Health Administration Press Marketing Manager at (312) 424-9470.

This publication is intended to provide accurate and authoritative information in regard to the subject matter covered. It is sold, or otherwise provided, with the understanding that the publisher is not engaged in rendering professional services. If professional advice or other expert assistance is required, the services of a competent professional should be sought.

The statements and opinions contained in this book are strictly those of the author(s) and do not represent the official positions of the American College of Healthcare Executives or of the Foundation of the American College of Healthcare Executives.

07   06   05   04   03   5   4   3   2   1

Library of Congress Cataloging-in-Publication Data

Schaffner, Julie W.
   Rx for the nursing shortage : a guidebook / by Julie W. Schaffner and
   Patti Ludwig-Beymer.
     p. cm.
   Includes bibliographical references and index.
   ISBN 1-56793-194-4 (alk. paper)
   1. Nurses—Supply and demand—United States. 2. Nursing—United States.
   I. Ludwig-Beymer, Patti. II. Title.
RT86.73 .S335 2003
331.12'9161073'0973—dc21

2002032897

The paper used in this publication meets the minimum requirements of American National Standard for Information Sciences—Permanence of Paper for Printed Library Materials, ANSI Z39.48-1984 ♾ ™

Acquisitions editor: Audrey Kaufman; Project manager: Joyce Sherman; Text and cover design: Matt Avery

Health Administration Press
A division of the Foundation of the
   American College of Healthcare Executives
1 North Franklin Street, Suite 1700
Chicago, IL 60606-4425
(312) 424-2800

This book is dedicated to my father, Everette J. Wine, who passed away suddenly while this book was in progress. May we all live every new day as he did ... with eagerness, with faith, with joy, and with love in our hearts.

—Julie Wine Schaffner

To my family and friends, who help me find balance, and to the heroic nurses of yesterday, today, and tomorrow, who are healthcare's greatest assets.

—Patti Ludwig-Beymer

Contents

Foreword

No ISSUE IS more critical to the future of healthcare in the United States than the perennial—and growing—shortage of skilled nurses. What makes the current state of shortage most troubling is that its causes are diverse and complex. No single treatment can cure the disease, nor can one individual, organization, or sector of our society alone solve this shortage.

The impact of the shortage is dramatic. California alone is expected to face a shortfall of approximately 25,000 nurses within the next several years. At Catholic Healthcare West (CHW), a 42-hospital system with facilities in California, Arizona, and Nevada, we are continually faced with about 1,000 nursing vacancies out of a total staff of 14,000 registered nurses. Every day our nursing managers must adapt to the current staffing level, in some cases forcing physicians and their patients to reschedule elective surgery to maintain our high standard of care for our patients. These problems are not unique to CHW. The crisis extends far beyond California, beyond the western states, and throughout the nation.

As healthcare professionals, we must address the nursing shortage systematically. Everyone from our government and community leaders to parents, educators, and families must get involved in the solution. The population of people who need nursing care is rising much faster than the population of nurses. Entry into college nursing programs tumbled 17 percent from 1996 to 2000; at the same time, those already in nursing careers reach closer to retirement or drop out of the profession because of burnout or other factors. At CHW, as at other healthcare organizations, we are working in high schools and colleges to help students learn about nursing careers. We participate in education loan forgiveness programs, and we are actively encouraging more people in our communities to choose—or return to—nursing careers.

These are all necessary steps toward solving the problems in the years ahead, but those of us who manage healthcare organizations today need to cope with our everyday staffing requirements. This is where authors Julie Schaffner and Patti Ludwig-Beymer are helping with their insight and perspective. Their book goes beyond the theory and into the practical reality of what it takes to recruit and retain the caring professionals we want at our patients' bedsides.

For many reasons, men and women are choosing careers other than nursing. The field of nursing is too often viewed as a "secondary" position in healthcare, playing a supporting role to physicians. Although they do provide support to their professional colleagues, nurses uniquely affect the delivery of healthcare at every step in the healthcare system. Nurses are entering a most challenging profession because they want to care for the sick and literally hold the hands of people at their darkest moments. Wages and benefits are important, but our nurses tell us they also want to continually provide better care, to learn new skills, and to find new techniques. As all of us should, today's nurses want a healthy balance between their dedication to work and their dedication to their personal lives and relationships. Providing this kind of work environment may be a tall order, but it is essential if we are to continue delivering on our healthcare mission.

Acting on this promise of a fulfilling employment experience is exactly what the authors help us do. Their guide to conducting an organizational climate assessment, for example, is an excellent starting point for healthcare organizations to identify obstacles to nursing satisfaction—which directly correlates to quality patient care. This is the same kind of internal evaluation that we conduct within CHW's hospitals to help us create programs like Career Ladder and Training Up, two of our continuing education incentive programs.

One of the more useful tools in this book is "100 Ways to Retain RNs," a handy checklist of specific measures that organizations can take *today* to help keep nurses fulfilled in their jobs and providing high-quality patient care. While some of the steps ought to be obvious (such as making sure that employees have professional development opportunities or thanking employees for special efforts), I am sure that every one of us will find at least a handful of new ideas on this list. One of my favorites on the list is number 73—pass out mini–stress relief kits to staff on an as-needed basis. Small efforts like this are often the most important ways we can tell people that we care about them and need them. At CHW, we put our values of collaboration, dignity, stewardship, excellence, and justice at the forefront of all of our activities. Small gestures recognizing and appreciating the contributions that nurses make to our healthcare mission go a long way toward keeping those nurses within the CHW family.

Also in the book is "100 Ways to Recruit RNs." This is a list of tangible steps that we can make today to reduce the nursing shortage—everything from letting job candidates know how we use advanced technology to improve their work environment, to creative work schedules, to mentoring programs with local high schools. Every one of these can work.

Read this book to learn practical steps to attract and preserve healthcare's valuable human assets. Nurses are the glue that holds our healthcare system together every hour, every day. They need to be recognized, rewarded, and valued. This book tells you how to do just that. As we implement programs to attract and retain nurses today, we will find ways to attract and retain nurses tomorrow.

Lloyd Dean
President and Chief Executive Officer
Catholic Healthcare West

Preface

WHEN WE WERE approached to write this book, we were very excited about the opportunity to be part of the solution to a nationwide care crisis that continues to escalate. We also had reservations, however, about our ability to balance our roles as wives, moms, and professionals while writing a book on a topic about which we are both passionate. We took the risk and in the process have learned a great deal from reading innumerable articles, books, and journals and from surfing the Internet.

We concluded that curing the nursing shortage is like losing weight—there is no magic pill or radical plan that will get you there. It requires a steady diet of consistency, steering a course and staying with it, using shortcuts for a very limited and targeted reason, and developing and using a support and networking structure.

Too often, the profession focuses on what is wrong with nursing instead of what is right with nursing. Staff members sometimes say, "I'm just a nurse," as if a nurse lacks value; the profession has a self-esteem crisis. Yet nursing is the glue that holds the healthcare delivery system together. It is the "can do" and "make do" profession—the RN always knows how to get things done—no matter what the odds. Without nurses, the American healthcare delivery system would not be the best in the world. Nursing is one of the most trusted professions, providing the caregivers whom patients and physicians rely on to care, heal, and be there at the beginning and end of life.

RNs work to promote health, prevent disease, and help families cope with illness. They educate and advocate for patients, families, and communities. Nursing is a difficult profession—one of self-sacrifice, hard work, long hours, erratic schedules, and challenging working conditions. Yet, it is also one of the most rewarding professions. Nurses make a difference, each and every day, and few professionals can say that.

This book was written to make a difference, too. Nurses dramatically affect the economics of healthcare, the overall quality of care, nursing-sensitive outcomes, prevention, adverse events, and patient satisfaction. To function effectively, healthcare organizations require an adequate number of well-educated professional nurses. Shortages in the supply of registered nurses have occurred frequently in the past; however, today's shortage is driven by a shift in the labor market that is unlikely to reverse in the short term.

Part I of this book, "A Nursing State of the Union," details the demographic characteristics, attitudes, expectations, and skills of the American nurse population. This introduction serves as a foundation for understanding the complexity involved in solving the nursing shortage crisis.

To meet the demand for RNs in this time of shortage, healthcare organizations must carefully plan and implement recruitment and retention policies. Parts II and III discuss strategies to enhance recruitment and retention efforts. Staff nurses as well as nursing leaders, including chief nurse executives, directors, managers, and supervisors, play key roles in ensuring the success of these strategies. Part II concludes with a "toolbox," "100 Ways to Recruit Nurses"; a similar toolbox, "100 Ways to Retain Nurses," follows Part III.

Part IV, "Leadership and Management: Strategies for Success," delves more deeply into the roles of the chief nurse executive and of senior and middle nurse managers. It also considers the new era of healthcare, and it concludes with the toolbox, "100 Ways to Lead."

Finally, Part V considers innovations in healthcare organizations that may lend potency to the prescription for solving the nursing shortage problem. This discussion focuses on the effect of magnet status designation as well as policy, regulatory, and legislative steps to alleviate the situation.

The nursing shortage is broad and complex; reversing it requires several different approaches. The challenges faced are formidable. However, with the talent of current and future nurses and with collaboration at all levels, they are surmountable.

We, the authors of this book, are nurses. We are not at the bedside, but we contribute to and affect nursing every day. We hope this book will help nurse leaders create the best professional practice environments that attract, recruit, and retain RNs. We want every RN to be able to say, "I am the nurse," with great pride and with the knowledge of the difference a nurse makes on the lives of those we serve.

Acknowledgments

SPECIAL THANKS TO MY HUSBAND, Tom, and our children, Kendell, Brian, and Lindsay, for their support; and to my secretary, Kathy, for the key role she played in this book project and the personal time she gave up to see it completed.

—*Julie W. Schaffner*

THANKS TO MY HUSBAND, Albert Sidney Beymer III, and our daughter, Theresa Beymer, for their unwavering encouragement, their willingness to eat take-out dinners, and their tolerance of my long hours on the computer; and to my mother and deceased father for always believing in me.

—*Patti Ludwig-Beymer*

PART I

A Nursing State of the Union

CHAPTER 1

Who Are the Nurses?

INTRODUCTION

Shortages in the supply of registered nurses (RN) have occurred frequently in the past, and a number of explanations have been proposed. Economists argue that shortages are related to lack of increase in real wages, an imperfectly competitive market, geographic distribution problems, or the delay between salary increases and ability to afford the education needed to enter the job market. Nursing leaders suggest that shortages are caused by a negative image of nursing, job dissatisfaction, downsizing, and restructuring (Seago et al. 2001). As early as 1915, leaders in nursing were concerned about the image of the profession. Since that time, countless studies have attempted to explain periodic nursing shortages (Friss 1993).

Whatever the reasons, today's registered nurse shortage is very real and very different from any experienced in the past. It stands in stark contrast to the oversupply predicted by the Pew Health Professions Commission (1995). Today's shortage is driven by a fundamental shift in the labor market that is unlikely to reverse in the near term (Buerhaus, Staiger, and Auerbach 2000a). It is characterized by fewer nurses entering the workforce, acute nursing shortages in some geographic areas, and a shortage of nurses prepared to meet patient needs in a changing healthcare environment.

To understand the current nursing shortage and plan effective strategies for recruiting and retaining nurses, this chapter provides basic information defining who the nurses are. The areas of discussion are as follows:

- An overview of the RN population is provided, with the current supply of nurses highlighted.
- Current and projected demands for nurses are summarized.
- Nursing specialty area shortages are highlighted.
- The use of international or foreign nurses is addressed.
- Nursing school enrollments and nursing faculty recruitment challenges are presented.

THE REGISTERED NURSE POPULATION

The National Sample Survey of Registered Nurses, conducted every four years since 1980, examines trends over time for RNs with an active license to practice in one or more of the U.S. states and the District of Columbia. The RN population increased by more than one million between November 1980 and March 2000. However, the years between 1996 and 2000 marked the slowest growth in the RN population. This slowdown reflects fewer new entrants to nursing as well as a larger number of losses from the nurse population than in previous years (Spratley et al. 2002).

The Current Supply of Nurses

Nursing is the largest healthcare occupation in the United States, with more than 2.5 million licensed registered nurses (U.S. Department of Labor 2002). The basic demographic characteristics of nurses are presented in Table 1.1. Most nurses are female, are married,

Table 1.1: Basic Characteristics of Registered Nurses

Characteristic	Statistic
Licensed registered nurses (number)	2,694,540
Female	94.6%
Average age	45.2 years
RNs under age 30	9.1%
RNs over age 50	30%
Employed in nursing	More than 75%
Employed full-time in nursing	71.4%
Employment setting	
Hospital	59.1%
Public/community health	18.2%
Ambulatory	9.5%
Nursing home and extended care facility	6.9%
Other (nursing education, state boards, health planning, insurance agencies, prisons)	6.3%

Source: Spratley et al. (2002).

and have children. However, the numbers of men and minorities entering nursing are increasing at a faster rate than the number of all registered nurses (MinorityNurse.com 2002). The number of African American, Asian or Pacific Islander, and American Indian or Alaskan Native nurses nearly tripled, and the number of Hispanic RNs doubled.

Nurses tend to commute, but not move, for a job. RNs are likely to work near the geographic area in which they were educated. Because the nursing workforce is less mobile than many other labor groups, regional geographic markets are an important factor in the workforce. In addition, female RNs tend to modify their work schedule to meet their family's financial and personal needs. For example, during economic downturns, the supply of RNs increases because nurses enter the labor market to replace their spouse's lost earnings (Seago et al. 2001).

The RN workforce is aging. Buerhaus, Staiger, and Auerbach (2000a) found that the average age of employed RNs increased by 4.5 years between 1983 and 1998. In contrast, the average age of the U.S. workforce as a whole increased less than two years during the same period. Similar aging trends have occurred in other positions traditionally dominated by women, such as teachers, social workers, secretaries, and hair stylists. Today, RNs in their 40s dominate the workforce, outnumbering RNs in their 20s by nearly 4 to 1. This contrasts with statistics from 1980, when the number of nurses in their 20s actually outnumbered the number of RNs in their 40s. In general, nurses work less and move away from the hospital setting as they age.

Although the numbers of minorities and men in nursing have increased recently, the percentage of each remains small. In particular, minority groups are poorly represented, as seen in Table 1.2. Considering these demographics, increasing retention efforts for middle-aged nurses and increasing recruitment for men and minorities is critical.

CURRENT AND PROJECTED DEMAND FOR NURSES

Job opportunities for RNs are expected to be very good. Employment of registered nurses is expected to grow faster than the average for all occupations through 2010, with a 21 percent to 35 percent increase in employment for RNs predicted. Faster-than-average growth will be driven by technological advances in patient care, which permit a greater number of medical conditions to be treated and an increasing emphasis on preventive care. Similarly, the number of older people, who are much more likely than younger people to need nursing care, is projected to grow rapidly. In addition, thousands of job openings will result from the need to replace experienced nurses who leave the profession, especially as the median age of the registered nurse population continues to rise (U.S. Department of Labor 2002). Based on projections from the Bureau of

Table 1.2: Race/Ethnicity of Registered Nurses Compared to the General U.S. Population

Race	% U.S. Population*	% Nurses**
Caucasian	75.1	86.6[†]
African American or Black	12.3	4.9[†]
Asian or Pacific Islander	3.7	3.7
Hispanic	12.5	2.0
American Indian or Alaskan Native	0.9	0.5
Other race	5.5	N/A
Two or more races	2.4	1.2

*Percentages add up to 112.4% because Hispanics may be of any race and are therefore counted under more than one category.

**Figures total less than 100% because some nurses chose not to report their racial/ethnic background.

[†]Non-Hispanic.

Note: N/A = not available.

Sources: Farella (2002); Hawke (2002).

Labor Statistics (U.S. Department of Labor 2002), one million new nurses will be needed by the year 2010.

Geography and Patient Demographics

Geography and patient demographics influence the supply of nurses. Some states report current and projected shortages of RNs, primarily because of an aging RN workforce and recent declines in nursing school enrollment, as seen nationally. Previous nursing shortages have been more intense in the Midwest and South than in the Northeast. Hospitals located in counties with a higher percentage of nonwhite residents had a higher probability of shortage. Nursing shortages were more likely in institutions with a higher share of patients insured by Medicaid. The insurance coverage of patients might reflect differences in the financial stability of hospitals or special challenges in caring for patients with Medicaid that affect the ability of the hospital to recruit RNs (Seago et al. 2001). These findings parallel physician shortages, which are more likely to exist in the South, in rural areas, and in areas of high minority populations (Council on Graduate Medical Education 1998).

Wages

Wage is not a significant predictor for RN shortage. Hospitals with a primary or total nursing care delivery model were less likely to report shortages when compared to hospitals that used team or functional nursing care delivery. Unit self-management and RN-physician collaborative committees were both associated with fewer RN shortages.

NURSING SPECIALTY AREA SHORTAGES

Whereas previous shortages affected nursing positions across the board, the current shortage is being felt most strongly in the critical care, emergency department, operating room, and pediatric intensive care areas. Only patients with the most serious conditions stay overnight, and these patients require a higher concentration of highly skilled nurses.

Major RN shortages in critical care units have been documented. Because intensive care units (ICU) have historically attracted younger RNs, the rapid decline in the number of RNs under the age of 30 in the workforce plays a role in explaining ICU shortages. Operating rooms and other perioperative areas such as postanesthesia care units are also having difficulty filling RN positions. This may be related both to the aging workforce and the decreasing number of diploma-prepared nurses. Nurses educated in diploma programs have historically been attracted to operating room specialties because they had extensive educational exposure to that area (Buerhaus, Staiger, and Auerbach 2000b).

Emergency departments (ED) are especially affected by decreased nurse staffing. According to a study released by the Center for Studying Health Systems Change (Brewster 2001), hospitals across the country are regularly diverting emergency department patients to other hospitals in the area. While ED diversions have always occurred seasonally, they are now a year-round problem.

Specific nursing skills are also in short supply. These skills include leading interdisciplinary teams, serving as patient educators, and managing care for patients across the continuum. Traditional hospital nursing positions are no longer the only options for employment. Opportunities for nurses in a variety of settings are abundant, particularly for nurses with advanced training and education. Unfortunately, many nurses have not been educated in these special skills and roles, which are typically learned at the baccalaureate and master's levels. The majority of practicing nurses in the United States have less than a baccalaureate education (Table 1.3).

INTERNATIONAL NURSES

Periodically, nations turn to immigration to satisfy labor needs, allowing people from other countries to enter and work with temporary, nonimmigrant visas. This strategy has been used periodically in the United States to resolve RN labor shortages (Glaessel-Brown 1998). Before 1965, selection of those eligible for immigration was based on the National Origins Quota System, which favored immigrants from the western hemisphere and set tight limits on immigrants from continents in the eastern hemisphere. The 1965 amendments to the Immigration and Naturalization Act of 1952 shifted priority to those who could demonstrate possession of valued skill, talent, knowledge, or experience (Xu, Xu, and Zhang 1999).

In response to a severe nursing shortage in the 1960s, the Immigration and Naturalization Act was again amended in 1970 to allow

Table 1.3: RN Education

Type of Education	Overall Basic Preparation (%)	1996–2000 Graduates (%)	Highest Level of Education (%)
Diploma in nursing	30	6	22
Associate degree	40	55	34
Baccalaureate degree	30	38	33
Master's or doctoral degree	—	—	10

Source: Spratley et al. (2002).

the U.S. entry of foreign registered nurses under the HIA category, which permits employment of foreign RNs in permanent jobs. Another nursing shortage in the 1980s resulted in passage in Congress of the Immigration Nursing Relief Act (INRA) of 1989 to create a special visa category for RNs. INRA allowed healthcare facilities access to foreign nurses while requiring employers to provide new protections to native RNs and reduce dependency on foreign-educated nurses. Unfortunately, during the time that INRA was in effect (1989–95), experienced foreign nurses took positions with entry-level salaries, which resulted in erosion of nurse wages. The Health Professionals Shortage Area Nursing Relief Act was introduced in 1997 after INRA expired.

Since it was enacted in 1995, the North American Free Trade Agreement (NAFTA) has permitted relocation of registered nurses from Canada. Although the types of workers admitted into the United States under NAFTA are not documented, Tabone (1999) indicates that a shortage of nurses in Canada may result at least partially from this agreement.

International nurses have never represented more than one percent of all nurses working in the United States; however, a few metropolitan areas have significant concentrations. For example, New York City officials reported that 20 percent of their nurses in the late 1980s were foreign born (Glaessel-Brown 1998). Most foreign nurses come from the Philippines, Canada, the United Kingdom, or India. Strong, institutionalized migrant networks exist. In addition, the General Accounting Office found that 85 percent of HIA temporary visa holders in healthcare filled permanent jobs (Glaessel-Brown 1998).

The nursing shortage has become a worldwide crisis. A return to using foreign nurses to resolve nursing shortages without developing an adequate workforce policy will result in continued cyclic registered nurse shortages and compound the international crisis (Tabone 1999). Major international newspapers report chronic nursing shortages that have resulted in cutbacks in services, shutdowns of some wards, postponement of new services, and delays in elective surgery (Grayson 2000). England, Canada, and the Philippines, once sources for nurse recruitment to the United States, are facing their own shortages. In fact, Canadian hospitals are aggressively recruiting U.S. nurses. Many countries, including Trinidad and Tobago and New Zealand, are moving to protect their nurses from recruitment (Grayson 2000).

Recently, the International Council of Nurses (ICN) Workforce Forum confirmed that both the supply and demand and the image and status of nurses are being seriously undermined. Working conditions threaten the health and safety of nurses and decrease the quality of care nurses are able to provide in many countries. Aggressively recruiting nurses from other countries may solve the recruiting nation's problems, but it only undermines the supply of nurses in the host nation.

With a worldwide nursing shortage, one country's gain is another country's loss. Therefore, it can only be addressed by working toward attaining an adequate, stable nursing workforce for the world. Working conditions must be addressed and the image of nursing enhanced so that people are attracted to the profession. ICN has drafted "Nurse Recruitment Principles: Ethical Framework" to raise awareness of the ethical issues surrounding international recruitment (Foley 2002).

NURSING SCHOOL ENROLLMENT

In all U.S. states and the District of Columbia, students must graduate from an approved nursing program and pass a licensing exam to obtain a nursing license. All states require periodic license renewal, which may involve continuing education. Three major educational paths are available to become a registered nurse:

1. associate degree in nursing (ADN)
2. diploma in nursing
3. bachelor of science degree in nursing (BSN)

There are 1,406 schools of nursing in the United States (Discover-Nursing.com 2002).

ADN programs, offered by community and junior colleges, take two to three years to complete. About half of the RN programs open in 2000 were at the ADN level (U.S. Department of Labor 2002). Some of the aging of the RN workforce has been attributed to the popularity of two-year associate degree programs during the 1980s. These programs tend to attract individuals in their middle to late 30s interested in a second career (Buerhaus, Staiger, and Auerbach 2000a). Diploma programs, administered by hospitals, also take approximately two to three years to complete. Only a small number of programs offer diploma-level degrees (U.S. Department of Labor 2002).

BSN programs, offered by colleges and universities, typically take four to five years to complete; however, some accelerated programs may be completed in as little as one year by students who enter with all of the prerequisite courses. According to the American Association of Colleges of Nursing (AACN), there were 84 accelerated baccalaureate programs in nursing in 2001, with an additional 23 programs planned (Howard-Ruben 2002). More than one-third of all programs in 2000 were at the BSN level. Nurses with a BSN degree are prepared to work in any setting, are considered better educated, and are in high demand. Many associate degree and diploma

Table 1.4: Average Age at Graduation (2000)

Type of Educational Program	Age
Diploma in nursing	30.8
Associate degree	33.2
Baccalaureate degree	27.5
All graduates	30.9

Source: Spratley et al. (2002).

nurses return to school to earn a baccalaureate degree. Some RN-to-BSN programs may be completed part-time; accelerated RN-to-BSN and BSN-to-MSN programs have also been developed. The average age at graduation of nursing students at the different levels is presented in Table 1.4.

Nursing school enrollment is cyclical, and for the past half-decade, it has been down. In 1995, for example, 96,610 people took the state nursing licensure exam. In 2000, only 71,475 people took the exam, a decline of 26 percent (Crow 2001). During the early 1990s, the numbers of nursing graduates increased in response to the shortage of the late 1980s and early 1990s. As a result, these graduates had an increasingly difficult time with placement. News of an oversupply of nurses in turn resulted in a decrease in enrollments in nursing schools by the late 1990s (Tabone 1999). Also, the misperception that fewer nurses would be needed in healthcare in the future was perpetuated. As a result, the number one challenge facing nursing schools nationally has been filling admission slots.

Following a six-year trend of declining enrollment in nursing programs, AACN reported an increase in enrollment in generic baccalaureate programs from 2000 to 2001 (Ulrich 2002). This change may reflect intensified and collaborative recruitment efforts and innovative and online programs. Nursing schools across the country have increased their recruitment efforts in response to the nursing shortage. Indiana University's School of Nursing successfully increased undergraduate enrollment by focusing on nursing as the gateway to a lifetime of career opportunities. Johns Hopkins University attributes its increase in enrollment to web site enhancements and the expansion of the student recruitment staff. In particular, second-degree students are actively recruited. In addition, the American Nurses Association has engaged in a major campaign to attract students to nursing. Obviously, these efforts need to be continued.

Nursing Faculty Changes

These success stories do not reflect the overall experience of most nursing programs. To complicate the situation further, a nurse educator shortage also exists. AACN reported a faculty vacancy rate of 7.4 percent; it found that most of the vacant positions entailed classroom and clinical responsibilities and almost all required or preferred a doctoral degree (Trossman 2002). Low salaries and lack of teaching experience are two reasons why filling open faculty positions is difficult.

Some of the factors behind the nurse educator shortage parallel the staff nurse shortage, including the aging workforce and salary issues. For example, the average age of full-time faculty in baccalaureate and graduate nursing programs is just over 50, and the average age of faculty holding doctorates is 55.9 (Trossman 2002). In addition, the average age of new doctoral recipients within nursing is 45 (National Research Council 1996). The aging of nursing faculty will affect the capacity of nursing schools to educate sufficient num bers of registered nurses to meet future demands. In terms of salary, nurses often make more money in clinical practice than in education. This is particularly true for advanced practice registered nurses (APRN). Faculty salaries at four-year programs have risen somewhat, but remain below APRN and managerial salaries.

Other factors contributing to the shortage are unique to nursing education, such as workload. Most universities have a mission for teaching, service, and scholarship. This leaves little time for faculty members to maintain their clinical practice and certification. Furthermore, universities primarily consider publications and grants as qualifications for tenured positions. Clinical expertise and practice are not a priority. In addition, nurses may be reluctant to pursue a doctorate if the degree does not provide sufficient return on investment in the long run.

Workload is also an issue for faculty in associate degree programs. Colleges tend to equate clinical rotations with science laboratory courses. They do not realize that overseeing students during clinical rotations is extremely labor intensive. This highlights the need to educate others about the education of nurses.

The faculty vacancy rate is likely to increase, as many faculty members are poised to retire with few replacements available. Within the next decade, some of the most experienced faculty members will be retiring. AACN considers the doctoral degree to be the most appropriate and desirable credential for nursing faculty. However, only 50 percent of all nursing faculty currently hold a doctoral degree (Howard-Ruben 2001). Although enrollment in doctoral programs has increased, relatively few nurses earn a doctorate, and competition for these students among schools of nursing is fierce. In addition, fewer than half of the students graduating from doctoral nursing programs plan to take a faculty role (Trossman 2002). Thus, the faculty shortage is likely to continue.

SUMMARY

Multiple sources suggest that the expected supply of nurses will not meet the future need. The aging of the nursing workforce is a major concern, as is the lag in minority representation. Unlike previous shortages, international nurses most likely cannot be recruited to alleviate the U.S. nursing shortage. Despite the positive regard with which the public generally holds nurses, general shortages and nursing subspecialty shortages, including faculty shortages, are predicted.

This chapter has described the population of the current supply of nurses, including specific demographic and education characteristics. The next chapter will address the movement of nurses, both within and outside of nursing.

REFERENCES

Buerhaus, P.I., Staiger, D.O., and Auerbach, D.I. 2000a. "Implication of an Aging Registered Nurse Workforce." *Journal of the American Medical Association* 283 (22): 2948–54.

———. 2000b. "Why Are Shortages of Hospital RNs Concentrated in Specialty Care Units?" *Nursing Economics* 18 (3): 111–16.

Brewster, L. 2001. "Emergency Room Diversion: A Symptom of Hospitals Under Stress." [Online article; retrieved Feb. 18, 2002.] Washington, DC: Center for Studying Health Systems Change. www.hschange.org.

Council of Graduate Medical Education. 1998. *Tenth Report: Physician Distribution and Health Care Challenges in Rural and Inner-City Areas.* Washington DC: U.S. Government Printing Office.

Crow, K. 2001. "Healing and Burnout, 12 Hours at a Stretch." *New York Times,* June 24. [Online article; retrieved July 20, 2001.] www.nytimes.com.

DiscoverNursing.com. 2002. "Nursing Programs." [Online article; retrieved Feb. 18, 2002.] www.discovernursing.com/program_search.asp.

Farella, C. 2002. "Erase the Hate: The Truth about Racism in Nursing." *Nursing Spectrum* 15 (41L): 8–9.

Foley, M.E. 2002. "President's Perspective: It's a Small World." *The American Nurse* Jan./Feb.: 4.

Friss, L. 1993. "Nursing Studies Laid End to End Form a Circle." *Journal of Health Politics, Policy and Law* 19 (3): 598–631.

Glaessel Brown, E.E. 1998. "Use of Immigration Policy to Manage Nursing Shortages" *Journal of Nursing Scholarship* 30 (4): 323–27.

Grayson, M. 2000. "Guard Your RNs!" *Hospitals & Health Networks* May: 22.

Hawke, M. 2002. "Mirroring Our Diversity." *Nursing Spectrum* 15 (41L): 10–11.

Howard-Ruben, J. 2002. "Second Degree Students Sprint to Nursing Careers." *Nursing Spectrum* 15 (31L): 8–9.

————. 2001. "Fewer Faculty Could Prove Hard Lesson for Nursing Profession." *Nursing Spectrum* 14 (16IL): 6–8.

MinorityNurse.com. 2002. "About MinorityNurse.com." [Online report; retrieved Nov. 1, 2002] www.minoritynurse.com/about.

National Research Council. 1996. *Survey of Earned Doctorates*. Washington, DC: National Research Council.

Pew Health Professions Commission. 1995. *Critical Challenges: Revitalizing the Health Professions for the Twenty-first Century*. San Francisco: University of California, San Francisco, Center for the Health Professions.

Seago, J.A., Ash, M., Spetz, J., Coffman, J., and Grumbach, K. 2001. "Hospital Registered Nurse Shortages: Environmental, Patient, and Institutional Predictors." *Health Services Research* 36 (5): 831–52.

Spratley, E., Johnson, A., Sochalski, J., Fritz, M., and Spencer, W. 2002. "The Registered Nurse Population: Findings from the National Sample Survey of Registered Nurses." [Online article; retrieved March 13, 2002.] Washington, DC: U.S. Department of Health and Human Services, Health Resources and Service Administration, Bureau of Health Professions, Division of Nursing. www.bhpr .hrsa.gov/healthworkforce/rnsurvey.

Tabone, S. 1999. "Thoughts on Nurse Shortages." *Texas Nursing* 73 (9): 4–5, 10–11.

Trossman, S. 2002. "Who Will Be There to Teach? Shortage of Nursing Faculty a Growing Problem." *The American Nurse* 1: 22–23.

Ulrich, B. 2002. "A Fresh Start." *Nurse Week* Jan./Feb.: 4.

U.S. Department of Labor, Bureau of Labor Statistics. 2002. *Occupational Outlook Handbook, 2002–2003 Edition*. [Online report; retrieved Feb. 18, 2002.] www.bls.gov/oco/home.htm.

Xu, Y., Xu, Z., and Zhang, J. 1999. "International Credentialing and Immigration of Nurses: CGFNS." *Nursing Economics* 17 (6): 325–31.

CHAPTER 2

Where Have All the Nurses Gone?

INTRODUCTION

The number of new nurses has declined in recent years; this is well-known. A fundamental shift occurred in the RN workforce during the last two decades. Explanations for the increasing age of RNs and the decreased numbers of nurses involve a combination of demographic, social, and educational forces. One factor, for example, is that young people are increasingly choosing other fields, such as information technology, that are perceived as more attractive than healthcare. Over the next decade, the RN workforce will continue to age, as the largest numbers of nurses will be in their 50s and 60s. The workforce will contract as these nurses retire (Buerhaus, Staiger, and Auerbach 2000).

This chapter attempts to answer the question, where have the nurses gone? It begins by summarizing the latest information on nursing morale and job satisfaction. It then identifies nonnursing career options, clinical practice changes in nursing, workplace injury or accident rates, and strategies for keeping nurses in nursing.

NURSING MORALE AND JOB SATISFACTION

In general, healthcare workers are more negative about their work than other U.S. workers. They express dissatisfaction about work and life harmony, career growth and development, compensation and benefits, and safety and security. One-quarter of healthcare workers indicate they experience fear, intimidation, and harassment in their work environment, and one-third of all healthcare employees say their managers do not meet their expectations. Top reasons healthcare workers give for seeking a new job include better pay, better work environment, better benefits, and advancement opportunities (Selvam 2001).

Negative Nurses

As the largest healthcare profession in the United States, nursing's voice is strongly heard and is equally negative. Most nurses participating in research conducted by Peter Hart Research for the Federation of Nurses and Health Professions (2001) mentioned poor morale as a problem. Furthermore, an international study found that low morale among hospital nurses is not unique to the United States. High percentages of nurses from the United States, Canada, England, and Scotland expressed dissatisfaction with their present job. The international study also measured nurse burnout and found that 43 percent of the U.S. nurses had high burnout scores, ranking higher than nurse burnout in Canada, England, Scotland, and Germany (Aiken et al. 2001).

The Peter Hart Research (2001) survey also reports the following findings:

- 21 percent of nurses now working are seriously considering leaving the profession within the next five years.
- Half of the nurses indicated they had thought about leaving nursing.

- Nurses under the age of 40 were nearly as likely to have thoughts about leaving nursing as their colleagues over the age of 50.

The nurses planned to leave not because they wanted to retire but because of working conditions. However, three-fourths of these nurses would consider staying if improvements were made. Increased staffing, better hours, and higher salaries were top reasons for staying (Peter Hart Research 2001). The research conducted by Aiken et al. (2001) in the United States, Canada, England, Scotland, and Germany showed similar findings, with 41 percent of the U.S. nurses dissatisfied with their jobs (Aiken et al. 2001).

Sources of Discontent

Of all the problems facing nurses, the number one issue identified by Peter Hart Research (2001) was staffing. Nurses described large patient loads, understaffing, not having enough time to spend with patients, and paperwork burden. Again, these findings are consistent with the international study (Aiken et al. 2001) findings in which nurses reported an increase in the number of patients assigned to them and insufficient staff to get the work done and provide high quality. In addition, Aiken and colleagues found that workforce management was also viewed negatively. Few U.S. nurses believed that administration listened and responded to nurses' concerns or that nurses' contributions to patient care were publicly acknowledged. Most indicated they had little opportunity for advancement and seldom participated in policy decisions. These workforce issues may be related to the elimination of some nurse manager and chief nurse executive positions (Aiken et al. 2001).

The importance of the nurse manager cannot be overestimated. The Nursing Executive Center found that more than 40 percent of nurses who were satisfied with their immediate manager considered leaving their current employer in the last year. For those nurses dissatisfied with their managers, that figure rose to 90 percent (Blizzard 2002). Assuming a competitive salary and similar environment, the research suggests that good managers are a key factor in retention. This book has devoted an entire section to the role of the manager in attracting and retaining staff. (See Part IV, "Leadership and Management: Strategies for Success.")

In addition, Peter Hart Research (2001) found that nurses view their jobs as becoming too stressful and physically demanding, and working conditions are perceived as worsening. However, the international study conducted by Aiken et al. (2001) suggests that not all aspects of hospital practice are unsatisfactory. U.S. nurses indicated that nurses are clinically competent and that physicians and nurses have good relationships, and salaries were viewed neutrally.

The Nursing Role

The international study (Aiken et al. 2001) carefully examined nonnursing tasks usually performed by nurses and nursing care interventions that were left undone during the last shift of the day. These findings are summarized in Table 2.1. Given the fact that nurses must leave essential interventions undone while performing nonnursing tasks, the conclusion that so many U.S. nurses are dissatisfied with their present job and plan to leave that job in the next year is not surprising (Aiken et al. 2001). In addition, a recent study conducted by PricewaterhouseCoopers for the American Hospital Association found physicians, nurses, and other staff members spend on average more than 30 minutes on paperwork for every hour of patient care. In the emergency department, every hour of patient care generates an hour of paperwork (Lewis 2001), allowing even less time for care and increasing frustration with the inability to find time to perform critical nursing activities.

Table 2.1: Nonnursing Tasks Performed and Nursing Care Left Undone

RNS who reported performing nonnursing tasks

Delivering and retrieving food trays	42.5%
Housekeeping duties	34.3%
Transporting patients	45.7%
Ordering, coordinating, or performing ancillary services	68.6%

RNS who reported necessary nursing interventions left undone

Providing oral hygiene	20.1%
Providing skin care	31.0%
Teaching patient or family member	27.9%
Comforting/talking with patients	39.5%
Developing or updating care plans	40.9%
Preparing patients and families for discharge	12.7%

Source: Aiken et al. (2001).

CAREER OPTIONS

Nonnursing Career Options

Declines in the number of nursing students reflect increased opportunities for women in other professions. For example, women interested in healthcare careers are more likely to enter medical school than in the past. Careers that have been historically male-dominated, such as business and law, are also more available to women. The dramatic changes in graduation of women in traditionally male-dominated programs of study over time are summarized in Table 2.2. In the 1950s and 1960s, when nursing schools successfully recruited students and the profession was expanding, fewer than 10 percent of business, dentistry, law, and medical students were female. A sharp shift occurred in the 1970s, with major increases in female enrollment seen in these programs.

Table 2.2: Percentage of Women Graduating in Male-dominated Professions, 1957–58 to 1997–98

Profession	1957–58	1967–68	1977–78	1987–88	1997–98
Business (baccalaureate degree)	7.5*	8.8	27.3	46.7	48.5
Business (master's degree)	3.6*	3.4	16.9	33.6	38.6
Computer and information science (baccalaureate degree)	N/A	N/A	25.7	32.4	26.7
Computer and information science (master's degree)	N/A	N/A	18.7	26.9	28.9
Dentistry	1.1	1.4	10.9	26.3	38.2
Law	2.9	3.9	26.0	40.5	44.4
Medicine	5.1	7.9	21.5	33.1	41.6

*1959–60.

Source: U.S. Department of Education, National Center for Education Statistics (2001).

Often, these professions are perceived as more prestigious, less stressful, and more accommodating to balancing work and family demands. In addition, the glamour and high pay of high technology are drawing potential and actual nurses away from nursing. Members of the Internet generation are not thrilled with the idea of work schedules that cover 24 hours a day and seven days a week.

Internal Migration of Nurses: Healthcare-related Options

The Balanced Budget Act of 1997, with its annual reductions in Medicare payments, affected the ability of hospitals to retain and provide financial incentives to nursing staff. These reductions have resulted in what many hospital nurses describe as job pressures, including increasing patient acuity, worsening nurse-to-patient ratios, less autonomy, and more administrative duties.

A significant number of licensed RNs no longer practice in the profession. In the United States overall, 18.3 percent of licensed registered nurses are not employed in nursing. The percentages of RNs not employed in nursing by state are presented in Table 2.3. An additional factor thought to contribute to the nursing shortage is part-time employment. In 2000, 28.4 percent of RNs worked part-time.

In addition to working part-time, nurses are choosing to work outside the hospital. Nonhospital jobs offer less shift work, more flexible hours, further skill development, equal or better pay, and lower levels of stress. Thus, growing numbers of nurses are leaving hospital staff nursing for other career opportunities. These include the following:

- case management for insurance companies
- home care
- outpatient services
- pharmaceutical research and sales
- healthcare product sales and marketing
- coordinating and monitoring clinical trials

Many of these opportunities, and others, are available as a result of an ongoing increase in nursing positions in home health, nursing homes, ambulatory care facilities, physician offices, and nontraditional healthcare settings. All of these are drawing nurses from healthcare delivery positions (Carpenter 2000).

Workplace Injury or Accident

Nurses do not expect to become sick or injured from conditions at work. However, work-related injuries and illnesses sometimes happen and may lead to nurses leaving the profession. According to the Occupational Safety and Health Administration (OSHA), an

Table 2.3: RNs Not Employed in Nursing in 2000 by State

State	%	State	%
Alabama	17.9	Montana	21.2
Alaska	16.7	Nebraska	11.6
Arizona	24.5	Nevada	19.8
Arkansas	19.5	New Hampshire	14.8
California	18.6	New Jersey	23.5
Colorado	20.9	New Mexico	13.0
Connecticut	18.3	New York	19.0
Delaware	14.7	North Carolina	16.8
District of Columbia	7.0	North Dakota	8.1
Florida	21.0	Ohio	17.7
Georgia	17.8	Oklahoma	15.9
Hawaii	16.7	Oregon	10.7
Idaho	18.3	Pennsylvania	25.3
Illinois	19.4	Rhode Island	15.7
Indiana	24.1	South Carolina	10.2
Iowa	11.6	South Dakota	11.2
Kansas	18.4	Tennessee	11.3
Kentucky	14.7	Texas	15.9
Louisiana	8.3	Utah	15.5
Maine	23.2	Vermont	15.5
Maryland	11.9	Virginia	24.2
Massachusetts	17.2	Washington	20.6
Michigan	21.3	West Virginia	12.4
Minnesota	14.2	Wisconsin	18.3
Mississippi	14.2	Wyoming	14.6
Missouri	13.9	**United States**	**18.3**

Source: Spratley et al. (2002, Appendix A, Table 39).

occupation injury is an injury that results from a work accident or a single exposure in the work environment, such as a needle stick or a fracture. An occupational illness is an abnormal condition or disorder caused by exposure to environmental factors associated with employment. Examples of occupational illnesses are allergic sensitization, repetitive muscle strain, and infection (Bain 1998).

A primary example of injury to nurses is related to back pain. Back pain affects more than 9 million people in the United States and accounts for 25 percent of all disability from work-related injuries. The incidence of back pain in nurses may be as high as 80 percent, accounting for more than 150 million lost work days for nurses annually (Smith-Fassler and Lopez-Bushnell 2001). Many of the injuries result from direct patient care activities, such as lifting (Retsas and Pinikahana 2000).

Nursing staff between the ages of 45 and 65 are at greatest risk for fall-related injuries, which indicates that general prevention strategies should focus on workers 45 years of age and older (Laflamme 1998). Little research has been conducted on occupational injuries in nurses as they age. However, it is well-known that humans are more susceptible to neck, back, and foot injuries and have a reduced capacity to perform some physical tasks as they age (Buerhaus, Staiger, and Auerbach 2000). Thus, all efforts to restructure patient care delivery must be ergonomically sensitive to older RNs.

KEEPING NURSES IN NURSING

Nurses themselves are a great source of ideas for helping solve the nursing shortage. The state of Wisconsin, for example, is requiring all of its 70,000 licensed RNs to complete an electronic survey to generate ideas for solutions. The goal is to seek information on why nurses leave the profession and what can be done to retain them. The survey is conducted as part of the nurses' license renewals. It was designed and supported by three state agencies and seven organizations representing nurses, including the Wisconsin Nurses Association, the Department of Health and Family Services, and the Wisconsin Health and Hospital Association (Price 2002).

Peter Hart Research (2001) asked nurses participating in its study how to improve retention and recruitment. Those who indicated they expected to leave nursing within the next five years identified strategies such as better staffing ratios, more patient time, more input into decisions, higher salaries, performance bonuses, flexible schedules, more part-time options, continuing education funds, and better health coverage. For themselves personally, nurses who expected to leave the profession within five years indicated they could be persuaded to stay with better pay, better staffing, better schedules, and more respect afforded them. Even former nurses indicated they could be pulled back into the profession with higher salaries, better staffing levels, and better schedules. Each of these factors is addressed later in this book.

SUMMARY

The number of new nurses has declined in recent years, and the size of the RN workforce is anticipated to be nearly 20 percent below projected needs by 2020. Nurses' morale and job satisfaction have clearly contributed to the widening gap between the number of existing practicing nurses and the number of nurses needed.

A variety of new career options are available to potential nurses, traditionally a largely female group. Over the past 30 years, the numbers of women educated in business, dentistry, law, and medicine have increased dramatically. In addition, changes in clinical practice have resulted in the movement of nurses into nonhospital positions or out of nursing entirely. Workplace injuries and accidents may also be contributing the migration of nurses.

This chapter has addressed a variety of factors that begin to answer questions related to the practice status of nurses. The next chapter in this section presents evidence of nurses' importance in healthcare.

REFERENCES

Aiken, L.H., Clarke, S.P., Sloane, D.M., Sochalski, J.A., Busse, R., Clarke, H., Giovannetti, P., Hunt, J., Rafferty, A.M., and Shamian, J. 2001 "Nurses' Report on Hospital Care in Five Countries." *Health Affairs* 19 (3): 43–53.

Bain, E.I. 1998. "Safe Nursing: Recognizing and Reporting Occupational Illness and Injury." *Massachusetts Nurse* 68 (4): 11.

Blizzard, R. 2002. "Shift Change: Where Did All the Nurses Go?" Gallup Tuesday Briefing, Feb. 2. [Online article; retrieved Feb. 18, 2002.] www.gallup.com/poll /tb/healthcare/20020205.asp.

Buerhaus, P.I., Staiger, D.O., and Auerbach, D.I. 2000. "Implication of an Aging Registered Nurse Workforce." *Journal of the American Medical Association* 283 (22): 2948–54.

Carpenter, D. 2000. "Going...Going...Gone?" *Hospitals & Health Networks* June: 32–42.

Laflamme, L. 1998. "Falls among Swedish Nurses and Nursing Auxiliaries: Types of Injuries and Their Relation to Age Over Time." *Work: A Journal of Prevention, Assessment & Rehabilitation* 10 (2): 147–55.

Lewis, C.B. 2001. "More than Money." *Hospitals & Health Networks* August: 56.

Peter Hart Research for the Federation of Nurses and Health Professions. 2001. "Survey: Nurse Shortage Will Be Worse than Current Estimates." Press release, April 19. [Online press release; retrieved Sept. 23, 2002.] www.aft.org/press/2001 /041901.html.

Price, C. 2002. "Short Staffing Watch." *The American Nurse* Jan./Feb.: 19.

Retsas, A., and Pinikahana, J. 2000. "Manual Handling Activities and Injuries Among Nurses: An Australian Hospital Study." *Journal of Advanced Nursing* 31 (4): 875–83.

Selvam, A. 2001. "The State of the Health Care Workforce." *Hospitals & Health Networks* 75 (8): 41, 43–43, 48.

Smith-Fassler, M.E., and Lopez-Bushnell, K. 2001. "Acupuncture as a Complementary Therapy for Back Pain." *Holistic Nursing Practice* 15 (3): 35–44.

Spratley, E., Johnson, A., Sochalski, J., Fritz, M., and Spencer, W. 2002. "The Registered Nurse Population March 2000, Findings from the National Sample Survey of Registered Nurses." [Online article; retrieved March 13, 2002.] Washington, DC: U.S. Department of Health and Human Services, Health Resources and Service Administration, Bureau of Health Professions, Division of Nursing. www.bhpr.hrsa.gov/healthworkforce/rnsurvey.

U.S. Department of Education, National Center for Education Statistics. 2001. *Digest of Education Statistics, 2000.* Washington DC: U.S. Department of Education.

CHAPTER 3

What a Difference
a Nurse Makes

INTRODUCTION

Nurses are a priceless healthcare resource that is not being protected or renewed. In *AMA News*, Michael Greenberg (2002) writes: "The U.S. Dept. of the Interior spends millions of dollars to protect our nation's endangered species. It writes long lists of plants and animals whose populations are dangerously low and hires scientists to figure out ways to increase their numbers. Too bad they haven't turned their attention to nurses." Greenberg goes on to describe how nurses create the protective environment needed by patients, providing knowledge, comfort, care, and compassion. Traditionally, nurses have been the interface between the hospital and the patients. While Greenberg acknowledges he has no solution to the problem, he believes that raising awareness is a good start.

This chapter begins by describing the positive public perception of nursing. It then briefly outlines the economic impact of recruiting for open nursing positions. Overall nursing quality and nursing-sensitive outcomes as well as other adverse events are presented as

Table 3.1: Public Perception of Honesty and Ethical Standards, by Profession (Percentage*)

Field	1997	1998	1999	2000	2001
Firefighters					**90**
Nurses			73	79	84
Druggists, pharmacists	**69**	**64**	69	67	68
Medical doctors	56	57	58	63	66
Clergy	59	59	56	60	64
College teachers	55	53	52	59	58
Dentists	54	53	52	58	56
Accountants				38	41
Bankers	34	30	30	37	34
Journalists	23	22	24	21	29
Members of Congress	12	17	11	21	25
Business executives	20	21	23	23	25
Lawyers	15	14	13	17	18
Car salespersons	8	5	8	7	8

*Percentage of respondents who indicate field has very high or high honesty and ethical standards.

Note: Bold type indicates top rating for that year.

Source: Moore (2001).

they relate to nurse staffing. Last, the impact of nursing on patient satisfaction is addressed.

THE PUBLIC PERCEPTION OF NURSES

The public perceives nurses very positively. The 2001 CNN/*USA Today*/Gallup poll indicates that 84 percent of the public rates the honesty and ethical standards of nurses as very high or high (Moore 2001). Results for several key groups are listed in Table 3.1. Of interest is that while both nurses and physicians rate very highly on the honesty and ethics survey, nurses have a significant edge.

AN ECONOMIC CASE FOR NURSES

Nursing positions are going unfilled nationally, with 11 percent of positions in hospitals documented as vacant. In 2001, 75 percent of hospitals reported that recruitment had become increasingly difficult over the past year. In addition, 39 percent of the hospitals reported that the cost of recruitment had increased. Recruitment dollars are being spent on general advertising, print ads, recruiters, job fairs, and Internet posting (Selvam 2001). A Gallup survey found that voluntary turnover of nurses was lower in hospitals with satisfied employees who were engaged in their work, resulting in lower recruitment costs and huge financial savings (Blizzard 2002).

Thus, successfully retaining staff is essential. Nurse managers are charged with developing personal relationships with staff members and fostering a positive work environment, actions critical for reducing turnover. Lower turnover will in turn lead to a more stable work environment and a better financial situation for the hospital.

THE IMPACT OF NURSING ON OVERALL QUALITY

Several studies have documented nurses' widespread concern that hospital nurse staffing is inadequate to provide quality care and protect the safety of patients (Shindul-Rothschild, Berry, and Long-Middletom 1996; Henry J. Kaiser Family Foundation 1999; Sochalski 2001). In one study, one in five nurses reported that the quality of nursing care in their unit during the last shift was only fair or poor. Nurses who rated the care on their unit as poor or fair also reported higher frequencies of medication errors, nosocomial infections, and patient falls with injuries (Sochalski 2001). The perception of quality of care was also troublesome in the international study conducted by Aiken and colleagues (2001), with only 35.7 percent of U.S. nurses agreeing that the quality of care on their unit was excellent and 44.8 percent indicating the quality of care in their hospital had deteriorated over the past year.

Internationally, physicians have expressed concern about the nursing shortage. A recent Commonwealth Fund survey of physicians in five countries found that physicians rank nurse staffing levels of hospitals as one of their most serious concerns in being able to provide high-quality healthcare (Aiken et al. 2001).

Nursing-sensitive Outcomes

A study commissioned by the American Nurses Association found a direct correlation between average nursing intensity weights, which measures the case-mix of patients, and average nursing hours and registered nursing hours per day. Furthermore, the study found a statistically significant inverse relationship between four patient incidents: as RN staffing increased, the number of pressure ulcers, non-community-acquired pneumonia, urinary tract infections, and postoperative infections decreased. Additionally, the study found statistically significant inverse relationships for staffing and length of stay; increased staffing was associated with decreased length of stay. Shorter lengths of stay and decreased morbidity strongly correlated to higher RN staffing (Blegen and Vaughn 1998). The Institute of Quality Healthcare (IQH), a consortium of 11 hospitals working to improve patients' quality of care, found that units with a staffing mix of up to 85 percent RNs had lower rates of medication errors per 10,000 doses and fewer patient falls (Blegen and Vaughn 1998).

A study cosponsored by the Health Resources and Services Administration Division of Nursing, Health Care Financing Administration, Agency for Healthcare Research and Quality, and National Institutes of Nursing Research of the National Institutes of Health found strong and consistent relationships between nurse staffing variables and five patient outcomes in medical patients: urinary tract infections, pneumonia, length of stay, upper gastrointestinal (UGI) bleed, and shock. In surgical patients, only the relationship between failure to rescue and nurse staffing was strong and consistent. Weaker evidence was found for urinary tract infections and pneumonias. Higher RN staffing was associated with a 3 to 12 percent reduction in the rate of outcomes potentially sensitive to nursing (OPSN), depending on the OPSN tested. Examples of OPSNs are given in Table 3.2. In addition, shifting from low to high values for all nurse staffing was associated with a 2 to 35 percent reduction in OPSN rates. For example, if nurse staffing shifted from low (first quartile) to high (third quartile) RN staffing, the models estimate a reduction in urinary tract infections in medical patients of up to 12 percent. If all nurse staffing (RN, licensed practical nurse [LPN] or licensed vocational nurse [LVN], and aide) were shifted from low to high, the estimated frequency of urinary tract infections in medical patients would decrease by up to 25 percent (Needleman et al. 2001). Results are summarized in Table 3.2.

In addition to rates of OPSNs, the results of the study provide evidence establishing the relationship between a number of patient outcomes and nurse staffing in acute care hospital inpatient units. The patient outcomes associated with nurse staffing are important. For example, length of stay applies to all inpatients, and reductions in length of stay decrease hospital costs as well as patient and family financial and psychological costs. Complications associated with nurse staffing involve large numbers of patients or are associated with substantial risk of death. Additionally, staffing shortfalls put patients at risk for dangerous, even deadly, complications.

Most recently, the *Journal of the American Medical Association* published an article describing research conducted by Dr. Linda Aiken, a nurse researcher, and colleagues. The study was designed to determine the nature of the relationship between registered nurses' workloads and patient outcomes. The researchers surveyed a variety of staff nurses and asked them how many patients they took care of at one time on the last shift worked. Responses were averaged for each hospital regardless of type of unit or shift to determine an institutional average. With a response rate of 52 percent,

Table 3.2: Association Between Nurse Staffing and OPSNs

Patient Outcome	Medical Patients			Surgical Patients		
	Relationship	Estimated Impact (% Decrease)		Relationship	Estimated Impact (% Decrease)	
		High RN Staffing	High All Staffing		High RN Staffing	High All Staffing
Failure to rescue	Inconsistent	—	—	Strong and consistent	4–6	2–12
Length of stay	Strong and consistent	3–6	3–12	None	—	—
Pneumonia	Strong and consistent	6–8	6–17	Weak	11	19
UGI bleed	Consistent	5–7	3–17	None	—	—
UTI	Strong and consistent	4–12	4–25	Some evidence	5–6	3–14

Note: OPSN = outcomes potentially sensitive to nursing; UGI = upper gastrointestinal; UTI = urinary tract infection.

Source: Needleman et al (2001, iii).

the average registered nurse–to-patient staffing level was 1 to 5.3 in the 168 hospitals included in the study. The study reported that surgical patient deaths or complications occur more often in hospitals where nurses care for more patients. Furthermore, job dissatisfaction is more likely in hospitals where nurses provide care to more patients (Aiken et al. 2002).

The Preventive Role of Nurses

Nurses also make a difference by providing physical and emotional patient safety. As amply documented in *To Err is Human* (IOM 1999), hospitalization is an inherent risk to a patient's safety. Nurses appear to play a strong role in prevention of complications related to the nosocomial hospital environment. Nurses also monitor the consequences of treatments, a patient's health status, the disease state or evolving condition, and the patients' ability to safely care for themselves (Stetler, Morsi, and Burns 2000).

To attain positive patient outcomes within a safety framework, nurses perform proactive behaviors to protect or rescue patients from both potential and actual negative events. For example, a nurse may detect and reverse an order error, thus preventing a complication. Similarly, when a nurse detects a complication, he or she initiates corrective actions to facilitate recovery and prevent further decline. Without appropriate and timely preventive behaviors, or without adequate nurse staffing and competency, nurses fail to rescue patients from at-risk or deteriorating conditions.

In a surveillance role, the nurse makes observations and assessments of the patient's condition and communicates as needed with medical colleagues. This surveillance role requires working with physicians for resolution and optimal prevention. Detection and prevention together reflect the nurse's focus on a patient's general function and physical safety. For example, the nurse monitors the patient after any procedure. Resolution and prevention together reflect the nurse's role of providing comfort and advocacy. In this capacity, a nurse may resolve a patient's conflict with other providers or manage a patient's symptom distress. These preventive activities performed by nurses serve to rescue patients and result in positive safety-related outcomes (Stetler, Morsi, and Burns 2000).

Adverse Events

Patients in intensive care units (ICU), as the name suggests, require substantial nursing care. Nurse staffing varies widely among ICUs, and the optimal nurse-to-patient ratio is unclear. However, recent research (Pronovost et al. 2001) suggests that the nurse-to-patient staffing ratio in the ICU may have an independent effect on the risk of postoperative complications in patients who have surgical repair of an abdominal aortic aneurysm. Mortality did not differ between the high nurse group (one nurse to one or two patients) and the low nurse group (one nurse to three or four patients). However, after adjusting for patient characteristics and hospital and surgeon volume, hospitals with fewer ICU nurses were more likely to have postoperative complications, particularly pulmonary insufficiency and reintubation. Even the addition of daily rounds by a critical care physician did not alter the risk for complications given the low nurse-to-patient ratio (Pronovost et al. 2001).

Kovner and Gergen (1998) found a significant inverse relationship between the number of registered nurses per patient day and urinary tract infections, pneumonia, thrombosis, and pulmonary compromise. The researchers estimated that one additional RN hour per surgical patient per day was associated with a 9 percent decrease in urinary tract infections and an 8 percent decrease in pneumonia. Blegen, Goode, and Reed (1998) found that having more unit RNs was associated with lower rates of decubiti, patient complaints, and nosocomial infections. In addition, research by Blegen and Vaughn

(1998) suggests that a higher nursing skill mix was associated with lower rates of medication errors and patient falls.

IMPACT OF NURSES ON PATIENT SATISFACTION

Patient satisfaction with quality of care is an important consideration in today's healthcare environment, with healthcare organizations motivated to satisfy and retain patients. Patient satisfaction is a complex phenomenon that requires patients to assess technical abilities and the cognitive and affective experience. It has been suggested that patients assess hospital care on affective aspects while assuming the technical aspects to be adequate (Vuori 1991). Previous research suggests that patients expect nurses to be capable, but are especially satisfied when nurses are caring, respectful, and communicative (Ludwig-Beymer et al. 1993).

Evidence suggests that nurses greatly affect patient satisfaction in a variety of ways. Nurses act as goodwill ambassadors and representatives for hospitals. They are viewed as responsible for day-to-day activities on a unit and are the main connection with patients (Abramowitz, Cote, and Berry 1987). In a study of 17,000 inpatients, nursing care accounted for 45 percent of variance in overall quality-of-care ratings (Carey and Seibert 1993). Another study found that low levels of nurse exhaustion were related to patient satisfaction, and high levels of nurse exhaustion were related to low levels of patient satisfaction. Patients on units where nurses found their work meaningful were more satisfied with all aspects of their hospital stay. Patients were less satisfied with their care on units where nursing staff felt more exhausted. In addition, patients were less satisfied with their care on units where nurses more frequently expressed intention to quit (Leiter, Harvie, and Frizzell 1998). This analysis suggests that patients' perceptions of the overall quality of care correspond to the relationship nurses have with their work. When nurses were unable to meet affective expectations, patients judged the quality of the entire hospital experience less favorably.

SUMMARY

Research suggests that nurses in hospital settings affect many aspects of care, including economics, overall quality, specific nursing-sensitive outcomes, other adverse events, and patient satisfaction. Much less is known about the effect nurses have in other practice settings, such as extended care and ambulatory care settings. More research is needed in all aspects of nursing practice.

Obviously, nurses cannot be viewed in isolation. They are part of a large interdisciplinary team needed for patient care. However, nurses clearly affect the health and well-being of patients in their care. Thus, our healthcare system requires a sufficient number of well-educated nurses. With this background understanding of the supply, demand, and importance of nurses, we move on to the "meat" of this book—strategies for recruiting and retaining these valuable healthcare providers.

REFERENCES

Abramowitz, S., Cote, A.A., and Berry, E. 1987. "Analyzing Patient Satisfaction: A Multianalytic Approach." *Quality Research Bulletin* April: 122–30.

Aiken, L.H., Clarke, S.P., Sloane, D.M., Sochalski, J.A., Busse, R., Clarke, H., Giovannetti, P., Hunt, J., Rafferty, A.M., and Shamian, J. 2001. "Nurses' Report on Hospital Care in Five Countries." *Health Affairs* 19 (3): 43–53.

Aiken, L. H., Clarke, S. P., Sloane, D. M., Sochalski, J., and Silber, J. H. 2002. "Hospital Nurse Staffing and Patient Mortality, Nurse Burnout, and Job Dissatisfaction." *Journal of the American Medical Association* 288 (16): 1987–93.

Blegen, M.A., Goode, C.J., and Reed, L. 1998. "Nurse Staffing and Patient Outcomes." *Nursing Research* 47 (1): 43–50.

Blegen, M.A., and Vaughn, T. 1998. "A Multisite Study of Nurse Staffing and Patient Occurrences." *Nursing Economics* 16 (4): 196–203.

Blizzard, R. 2002. "Shift Change: Where Did All the Nurses Go?" Gallup Tuesday Briefing, Feb. 2. [Online article; retrieved Feb. 18, 2002.] www.gallup.com/poll/tb/healthcare/20020205.asp.

Carey, R.G., and Siebert, J.H. 1993. "A Patient Survey System to Measure Quality Improvement: Questionnaire Reliability and Validity." *Medical Care* 31: 834–845.

Greenberg, M. 2002. "Hailing One of Health Care's Priceless Resource—Nurses." *American Medical News* Jan. 28. [Online article; retrieved Feb. 18, 2002.] www.ama-assn.org/sci-pubs/amnews/amn_02/edca0128.htm.

Henry J. Kaiser Family Foundation and Harvard School of Public Health. 1999. "1999 Survey of Physicians and Nurses." [Online article; retrieved Feb. 5, 2002.] www.kff.org.

Institute of Medicine. 1999. *To Err is Human: Building a Safer Health System,* edited by L. T. Kohn, J. M. Corrigan, and M. S. Donaldson. Washington, DC: National Academy Press.

Kovner, C.T., and Gergen, P.J. 1998. "Nurse Staffing Levels and Adverse Events Following Surgery in U.S. Hospitals." *Image* 30 (4): 315–21.

Leiter, M.P., Harvie, P., and Frizzell, C. 1998. "The Correspondence of Patient Satisfaction and Nurse Burnout." *Social Science Medicine* 47 (10): 1611–17.

Ludwig-Beymer, P., Ryan, C.J., Johnson, N.J., Hennessy, K.A., Gattuso, M.C., Epsom, R., and Czurylo, K. 1993. "Using Patient Perceptions to Improve Quality Care." *Journal of Nursing Care Quality* 7 (2): 42–51.

Moore, D. W. 2001. "Firefighters Top Gallup!" Honesty and Ethics List, Gallup News Service. [Online article; retrieved Feb. 18, 2002.] www.gallup.com/poll/releases/pr011204.asp.

Needleman, J., Buerhaus, P.I., Mattke, S., Stewart, M., and Zelevinsky, K. 2001. "Nurse Staffing and Patient Outcomes in Hospitals." Final Report. Washington, DC: U.S. Health and Human Services, Health Resources and Services Administration.

Pronovost, P.J., Dang, D., Dorman, T., Lipsett, P., Garrett, E., Jenckes, M., and Bass, E.B. 2001. "Intensive Care Unit Nurse Staffing and the Risk for

Complications after Abdominal Aortic Surgery." *Effective Clinical Practice* 4 (5): 199–206.

Selvam, A. 2001. "The State of the Health Care Workforce." *Hospitals & Health Networks* 75 (8): 41, 43–46, 48.

Shindul-Rothschild, J., Berry, D., and Long-Middletom, E. 1996. "Where Have All the Nurses Gone? Final Results of Our Patient Care Survey." *American Journal of Nursing* 96 (11): 24–39.

Sochalski, J. 2001. "Quality of Care, Nurse Staffing, and Patient Outcomes." *Policy, Politics, & Nursing Practice* 2 (1): 9–18.

Spratley, E., Johnson, A., Sochalski, J., Fritz, M., and Spencer, W. 2002. "The Registered Nurse Population March 2000, Findings from the National Sample Survey of Registered Nurses." [Online article; retrieved March 13, 2002.] Washington, DC: U.S. Department of Health and Human Services, Health Resources and Service Administration, Bureau of Health Professions, Division of Nursing. www.bhpr.hrsa.gov/healthworkforce/rnsurvey.

Stetler, C.B., Morsi, D., and Burns, M. 2000. "Physical and Emotional Safety. A Different Look at Nursing-sensitive Outcomes." *Outcomes Management for Nursing Practice* 4 (4): 159–66.

Vuori, H. 1991. "Patient Satisfaction—Does It Matter?" *Quality Assurance in Health Care* 3: 183–89.

Appendix 3.1: Employed Nurses per 100,000 Population by State, 2000

State	Number of Nurses	State	Number of Nurses
Alabama	766	Montana	812
Alaska	596	Nebraska	958
Arizona	628	Nevada	520
Arkansas	701	New Hampshire	916
California	544	New Jersey	800
Colorado	737	New Mexico	656
Connecticut	942	New York	843
Delaware	936	North Carolina	858
District of Columbia	1,675	North Dakota	1,096
Florida	785	Ohio	882
Georgia	683	Oklahoma	635
Hawaii	703	Oregon	793
Idaho	636	Pennsylvania	1,010
Illinois	819	Rhode Island	1,101
Indiana	761	South Carolina	728
Iowa	1,060	South Dakota	1,128
Kansas	885	Tennessee	872
Kentucky	833	Texas	606
Louisiana	834	Utah	592
Maine	1,025	Vermont	957
Maryland	856	Virginia	711
Massachusetts	1,194	Washington	738
Michigan	798	West Virginia	858
Minnesota	957	Wisconsin	893
Mississippi	750	Wyoming	780
Missouri	960	**United States**	**782**

Source: Spratley et al. (2002, Appendix A, Table 39).

PART II

Recruitment Strategies that Work

CHAPTER 4

The Recruitment Road Map

INTRODUCTION

A collaborative planning process between nursing, human resources, marketing, and public relations departments is essential in developing and executing an effective nursing recruitment plan. The format you select may be found in strategic planning books, adapted from internal planning processes, or customized to your organization's needs and developed using any format that meets your needs and is easy to understand. A template is used to demonstrate one approach that has been used successfully to assess recruitment strategies.

This chapter will demonstrate a process that identifies goals and objectives; includes and defines SWOT analysis; identifies recruitment tips, sources, and resources; and helps you evaluate your new plan. A SWOT analysis case study and sourcing calendar job aid are presented to illustrate several ideas discussed in this chapter.

Workforce-needs planning for the short and long term will be addressed, along with the actual recruitment process. Steps to assess your effectiveness and monitoring indicators will be provided. Supplying practical ways to plan, evaluate, and implement the recruitment process is the focus of this chapter.

DEFINING THE GOALS AND OBJECTIVES OF THE RECRUITMENT PLAN

Developing goals and objectives guides your recruitment plan and keeps it focused on what you need to accomplish, as well as serving as a communication vehicle. Review these questions:

What is the goal of the recruitment plan?
To ensure a continuous supply of RNs by using a proactive approach to recruiting for the short and long term.

What are the objectives of the recruitment plan?

1. to complete a SWOT analysis of internal and external effectiveness
2. to evaluate workforce needs for the next three years
3. to identify traditional and nontraditional RN recruitment sources
4. to develop an effective recruitment process that is consistent for all recruiters
5. to develop an annual sourcing calendar
6. to develop a monitoring process

Complete a SWOT Analysis

A preliminary step in identifying your recruitment strategy and developing a plan is to complete a SWOT analysis. This analysis is an effective way to identify the strengths and weaknesses of your healthcare facility and provides a way to examine opportunities and threats. It will also enable you to clearly see the changes that need to be made in your organization to increase recruitment effectiveness. Internal information is used for strengths and weaknesses; opportunities and threats are gathered from the external environment:

Strengths: What are your advantages? What do you do best?
Weaknesses: What can be improved?
Opportunities: What are the current trends in recruitment?
How can you benefit from them?
Threats: What obstacles do you face? What is the
competition doing?

Brainstorming is the best way to accomplish the SWOT analysis, and utilizing different target audiences will strengthen the analysis. This technique involves having each participant share ideas, without critique, and placing all those ideas on a flip chart as they are suggested. Senior nursing leadership, middle managers, and staff RN groups should provide input. Brainstorming has the added advantage that it is a visible way to involve staff in the process and demonstrate your commitment to filling nursing vacancies. Keep the SWOT brainstorming group to ten or fewer people and be very clear on the purpose of the brainstorming—to analyze the current recruitment process.

Strengths. Identify the strengths of your healthcare facility and nursing department, with a focus on those factors that are important to staff recruitment. Such factors as quality of work life, clinical advancement, national hospital recognition, percentage of BSN- and MSN-prepared nurses within the organization, salary and benefits, RN staff-to-patient ratios, vacancy and turnover rates, nursing governance, staff satisfaction, physician support, technology enablers, and management support should be considered. What attracts RNs to your facility? What do you offer that is unique? For example, tuition reimbursement and flexible staffing are strengths that can be identified.

Weaknesses. Identify weaknesses of your recruitment strategy and weaknesses within your facility that will affect effective recruitment. How is nursing perceived? How are new staff treated? What materials do you use for recruitment? For example, lack of tuition reimbursement, too few recruiters and/or a lack of competency of recruiters, an inadequate budget, lack of a web-based strategy, lack of innovative tactics, and lack of an advertising strategy are fundamental weaknesses.

Opportunities. Identify opportunities for your recruitment planning, capitalize on the weaknesses of your competitors, and evaluate your internal opportunities that have not been realized. Such opportunities may include implementing a web-based strategy, developing a recruiter-training program, identifying innovative tactics in the marketplace, and marketing positive attributes of the facility. Consideration should be given to the development of a strategy that cannot be replicated by your competitors, such as being the only organization in your market that has achieved magnet status from the American Nurses Credentialing Center, or the only employer that offers career paths and transfer opportunities within a healthcare system or that allows for professional growth and development without changing employers.

Threats. Marketplace and internal threats should be considered. A competitor analysis is particularly beneficial and can be obtained by your marketing department or from a variety of sources, including telephone calls to competitor organizations, salary data from local healthcare organizations, a review of advertisements, and information from former employees. What are the threats to effective recruitment that will affect your success? Higher salaries and benefits at competing healthcare organizations, substandard working conditions, lack of technology, lack of nursing participation in decision making, lack of flexible schedules, and lack of adequate staffing are factors to be considered. High nursing turnover and vacancy rates should also be considered as a threat to future success.

A SWOT analysis enables your nursing division and its leadership to critically evaluate the recruitment process in an objective way. It can also be used to evaluate a single clinical unit such as oncology, or a nursing section such as critical care, that is facing significant recruitment challenges related to turnover, service expansion, and supply and demand issues.

A hospital-based nursing division SWOT analysis is presented in Figure 4.1 and illustrates the use of this technique.

Figure 4.1: SWOT Analysis

A case study

Faith General Hospital, a 331-bed hospital in a mid-size midwestern town embarked on a recruitment planning process. Two other hospitals are in the same city. The RN vacancy rate at Faith General is 7% and the turnover rate is 9%. The hospital has never had a recruitment problem before.

The hospital's chief nursing executive started the initiative by holding a full-day nursing retreat with the nursing directors, the director of public relations, and the director of human resources. Several RN recruiters were also present. A SWOT analysis was completed and the group found the results to be compelling.

Strengths
1. Excellent working relationship between human resources, public relations, and nursing
2. Hospital named as top employer in area for five years
3. Financial strength of hospital is best in market
4. Flexible schedules offered to RNS
5. Stable management
6. Strong physician support for nursing
7. High percentage of BSN-prepared RNS employed
8. Clinical advancement program in place
9. Faith-based and values-driven organization
10. Excellent continuing education and clinical support for staff

Weaknesses
1. Inadequate recruitment budget
2. Too few recruiters
3. Few enablers for nursing such as automation
4. Wages are lagging behind competitors
5. Inadequate electronic capabilities internally
6. No "refer a friend" program
7. Lack of awareness of nursing shortage by governance and CEO
8. Lack of recruitment and retention committee

Opportunities
1. Capitalize on difference in being a faith-based, values-driven organization
2. Utilize expertise of public relations and human resources for strategy development **(continued)**

Figure 4.1 *(contined)*

3. Evaluate salary structure and identify ways to address within budgetary parameters
4. Implement "refer a friend" program
5. Build on evolving technology strategy to enhance electronic capabilities
6. Promote value of clinical advancement program
7. Utilize physician leadership to promote the value of nursing
8. Establish internal recruitment and retention committee and develop strategy
9. Build on reputation for clinical excellence

Threats
1. Two competitors recently increased wages, making their wages 3 percent higher than Faith General's
2. For-profit surgery center and rehabilitation center are being built in area and are offering hiring bonuses and premium pay rates
3. Academic center 30 miles away has targeted your city for RN recruitment
4. Physicians' offices are offering similar wage packages andbetter hours
5. Faith General's most successful RN recruiter and several staff have been hired by a competitor
6. Local nursing school is closing after academic year

After the preliminary SWOT analysis was completed, the results were analyzed and the information was used to develop a plan.

The strengths were evaluated to take advantage of the opportunities. A strength is that the organization is faith-based and values-driven, and the resulting opportunity is to build on that reputation when recruiting RNs. A strength that can be used to reduce the threat of wage increases by competitors is to build on Faith General's clinical advancement program and flexible schedules because these benefits are very important to nurses.

Weaknesses can be turned into opportunities. Governance and the CEO can be educated about the nursing shortage and a request made to increase wages to the level of the competition, with statistics presented on how many staff were lured away by higher wages. Weaknesses can also be used to counteract threats. The competition's hiring of the best recruiter is viewed as a threat. Having too few recruiters is a weakness. The strategy becomes one of hiring the best recruiter in the field to counteract both a weakness and a threat that has been identified.

Determine Workforce Needs

By determining workforce needs, you will be able to proactively plan for those needs, both for the present and and the future. A needs assessment, along with long- and short-term strategies, will ensure your RN workforce needs are met.

Complete a Needs Assessment

First, an inventory and analysis should be done on current and projected skills and needs. An assessment of those tools should follow and should include the feasibility of redeployment of existing personnel to other departments or work sites. Needs should be quantified as much as possible, and assessments should be completed annually. Questions to consider include the following:

What new services or additional beds will require more RNs? Identify new services such as a pediatric cardiovascular program or the addition of new critical care beds. Consider any new ambulatory services that will require more RNs in the next year. Conversion of beds, such as from psychiatry to medical, will change the type of RNs needed. Take this into consideration, especially if retraining is required.

What skills and types of personnel are needed now and in one year? Consider the need for enhanced telemetry skills or for services you are transitioning to a different level of care, such as from inpatient child psychiatry to outpatient child psychiatry. Be specific about competencies, knowledge, special skills, education, and experience levels you are seeking.

Which positions can be filled within the hospital or hospital system? Determine if you can grow your own staff internally, for example, by hiring unlicensed assistive workers when they are nursing students and helping them transition to the RN role in your facility after graduation. Evaluate whether you can enhance the competency of nonspecialty RNs to help them move into a critical care role.

What positions will be the most challenging in terms of recruitment? Positions in areas like adult and pediatric critical care are often the hardest to fill. These should be placed on your "hot list" or "critical to fill" list. Different strategies may be needed for these efforts; for example, hire-on bonuses may be required.

What positions are best for targeted subgroups (e.g., Net generation, generation X, re-entry RNs, second-career RNs)? Learn from experience: what positions seem to work best in retaining target populations? For example, a re-entry RN may be better suited for a job in the medical/surgical department or a less intense environment for at least the first year. A new graduate may be better suited for a job that offers cross-training in a formal internship program. A second-career RN may add value in the arenas of education or quality improvement or may serve as a mentor in a clinical area.

Ask the following questions related to your personnel planning needs:

- *What?* Again, be specific about the skills, knowledge, abilities, experience, and education requirements you are seeking. Identify and quantify any changing needs, such as 10 percent more pediatric RNs and 20 percent fewer psychiatry RNs.
- *How many?* What is the recruitment goal by job class or job in terms of numbers? Look at turnover in the past year and additional needs because of new services. You may target 10 new graduates for medical positions and 20 pediatric RNs after opening a new unit.
- *Where?* What departments have the most openings? Are certain shifts difficult to fill? Which ones? For example, medical oncology may have a critical need on the night shift, requiring four more RNs.
- *When?* Define needs for the next 12 months. Do your planning as part of the budget cycle.

Many strategies are available for workforce planning/strategic staffing needs. Strategies can be divided into those that meet short-

and long-term needs; both are important to the organization's overall success. The nursing shortage is not likely to end for many years to come; thus, the organization that is proactive in identifying and implementing strategies to meet its needs will continue to prosper. Proactive planning is a key factor in your organization's success.

Think about strategies for the short term as those that can be implemented in one year or less; long term should be greater than one year, with the end point (e.g., one to three years) defined by your organization. This time frame is dependent on how severe the shortage is in your geographic area and how far in advance your organization plans. Evaluate what has been successful in the past and what needs to be improved.

Identify Long-term Strategies for Planning Purposes

Student Awareness Tactics

Student awareness tactics include school outreach activities, provision of materials such as MTV-like videos and age-appropriate materials, summer nursing camps, shadowing programs (in which students "shadow" or follow a nurse around for a specified period of time; this exposure provides the chance to see a real-life nurse in action in a particular setting), and work/study programs with local high schools.

> **Planning tip:** Develop a student awareness tactic, assign accountability, define the timeline, and identify budgetary requirements.

Loan and Scholarship Tactics

Loans and scholarships require advance planning to identify and procure funding sources, develop criteria for eligibility, prepare marketing materials, and complete finance and legal department reviews.

> **Planning tip:** Consider whether you will seek internal or external funding and the timeline for procurement of funding. Assign accountability for the tactic. Ensure that a cost-benefit analysis is completed and requirements for eligibility and loan payback are evaluated.

RN Student Rotations, Internships, and Summer Employment Tactics

Any long-term plan requires consideration of student rotations into the clinical areas of your facility, including electives in areas like the operating room and critical care, development of new graduate internships, and summer employment programs for student RNs.

> **Planning tip:** Assign your education department to this tactic and have it target the schools and clinical rotations you wish to have or enhance, assign curriculum development for a nursing internship, and identify budgetary and human resource needs that this tactic requires.

Identify Short-term Strategies for Planning Purposes

Short-term planning enables you to meet workforce needs for the year and keeps you focused on activities to meet your more immediate staffing demands.

Develop a Sourcing Calendar

Short-term planning requires you to assess how you will recruit in the coming year and what fiscal and human resources will be required. A monthly calendar of recruitment activities is helpful in planning for staff and operating expenses. The purpose of the calendar is to ensure that you plan for the resources you need while doing the budget for the year and document what you want to do, obtain support for your plans on the front end, and are able to implement them throughout the year.

Mailing lists, job fair fees, advertising fees, agency recruiting fees, and internal refer-a-friend bonuses are effective in short-term recruiting and need to be planned for to ensure they can be implemented. A sourcing calendar, such as the one shown in Figure 4.2, can be used for planning and budgeting for the year and provides for a recruitment activity each month.

Identify Recruitment Sources and Resources

Never overlook any potential sources to tap for your recruitment plan. Identify all such sources as part of your plan. If the sources need to be researched, make this a tactic in itself and leave the specific sources off the plan. Sources will, in turn, generate leads. Several to consider include:

- newspaper and print ads
- the Internet
- professional publications
- posting services through specialty organizations
- feedback from current employees
- laid-off employees from other healthcare organizations
- current employee refer-a-friend program or word of mouth
- sourcing specialists or recruiters who call the workplace or home of prospective employees
- continuing education events or professional meetings
- recruiting booths at community health events or fairs
- external recruiters working on commission
- schools of nursing

Figure 4.2: Sourcing Calendar

January	February	March	April
Movie "trailers"	Nursing Spectrum advertising for target areas	RN student open house	Billboard on interstate
Open house held by clinical managers			Electronic job fair
			Career fair
May	**June**	**July**	**August**
Electronic postcard to all RNS in primary and secondary markets	Critical care convention for recuitment	Radio campaign	Nursing Spectrum full-page ad
		Critical care open house	
New graduate direct mail	RN open house	RN hero and heroine stories in paper	Focus groups with agency and PRN RNS
	Campaign for part time to full time		
September	**October**	**November**	**December**
High school presentations	Radio ads	Electronic job fair	Call all qualified staff who have left in last six months for re-hire
Direct mail campaign for "hard to fill" areas	On-site rehabilitation conference for recruitment	Direct mail campaign	
		Career pathing event	Wine and cheese party for student RNS
Refer-A-Friend Month			

Why make this part of the plan? Some of these efforts require funding and lead time, and proactive planning will help you get a jump start on the year's recruitment endeavors.

In recruitment, resources must also be clearly identified to implement your plan. A number of key resources should be included:

- *Full-time recruiters.* How many do you need? What is the salary?
- *Advertising and marketing budget.* Identify what you will spend based on the plan; be sure to include costs for advertising, postage, brochures, lists, and journal and Internet advertising for the year.
- *Printing.* Determine the cost of direct mail, brochures, letters to employees with recruitment news, newsletters, cafeteria tents, postings, and so forth.
- *Events.* Determine the cost of booths, refreshments, media for posters and other materials, and any personnel travel.
- *Sourcing costs.* Sourcing specialists will make cold calls and do research for you on hard-to-fill positions and can be hired or used on a temporary basis. Identify the cost of this resource if you plan to use it.
- *External agency costs.* Project external recruitment costs at approximately 30 percent of salary or the cost of buying out any agency contracts. Look at cost effectiveness of this tactic.
- *Software and hardware.* Plan for any recruitment software and hardware purchases, upgrades, maintenance contracts, or technical support that will be required.

THE RECRUITMENT PROCESS

Most hospitals face significant recruitment challenges, which in turn affect patient and RN satisfaction and the ability to provide adequate staffing. The goal is to generate more leads that become employees, with fewer resources, in less time. Although this goal is daunting, a task-oriented recruitment process can be turned into an effective recruitment business in a number of ways.

The best use of a recruiter's time is with qualified and interested candidates, yet paperwork and data entry often consume more time. Automation of the process can improve *efficiency* but not necessarily *effectiveness*. To make the process work effectively, an analysis of each step of the recruitment cycle should be completed. Steps to a successful recruitment program include the following:

1. Define each step of the recruitment process so that it is easily understood.
2. Ensure appropriate personnel utilization and training.
3. Ensure effective generation of leads through sourcing.
4. Provide a consistent and standardized interviewing and selection approach.
5. Ensure appropriate tracking and follow-through during the process.

Because the process itself can affect whether candidates choose your facility, each step is described in detail below.

Define Each Step of the Recruitment Process so It Is Easily Understood

Use a flow chart to identify each step in the process, who is involved, and how long it takes. Usually, there is ample opportunity for improvement. Start with the application process and end with the candidate hired. Involve all staff who are part of the process in the activity. Figure 4.3 demonstrates a recruitment process flow chart.

Ensure Appropriate Personnel Utilization

Your organization needs to determine if the recruiters should be RNs. This is dependent on your budget, available resources, and whether

Figure 4.3: Steps in the Recruitment Process

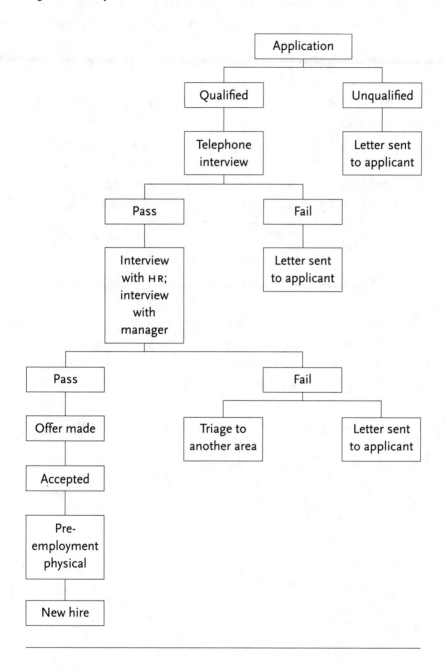

the focus is on nursing only or includes other, nonnursing areas. Once this is determined, the organization needs to assess the support structure. A recruitment assistant may be a cost-effective adjunct to the recruitment staff and will often improve the productivity of the recruiter by helping to generate leads, completing paperwork, making candidate appointments, ensuring that all logistical details are completed, and ensuring rapid-cycle turnaround. This allows the recruiter to spend the majority of his or her time interviewing and recruiting, given that it takes approximately ten leads to generate a hire. The recruitment assistant also ensures all post-hire processes are completed. Each recruiter and assistant should be assigned to a group of nursing units in a large facility to build trust and rapport with the managers and establish accountability.

Ensure Effective Generation of Leads: Sourcing Candidates

Recruitment sources were identified as a way to generate leads as part of workforce needs planning. For the process itself, a continuous supply of leads gained through various sources is a critical success factor. The following sources can be used to generate leads:

- advertising (print ads, radio spots, TV spots, billboards)
- employee referral programs
- trade shows, publications, and job fairs
- specialty nursing conferences
- national nursing conventions
- direct mail
- Internet
- intranet
- "hot jobs" profiling
- e-mail
- community events
- educational offerings open to the public

Provide a Consistent and Standardized Interviewing and Selection Process

Each recruiter should have a consistent approach to each aspect of the recruitment process related to interactions with candidates. Scripts are recommended to ensure consistency and efficacy in the process from start to finish. They should focus on making the candidate feel at ease and important. Part of the job of the recruiter is telling about the position and "selling" the healthcare facility and the department.

A script should be used to screen the candidates to ensure job skills are present. In addition, questions to assess a cultural fit with the organization should be included. Questions may relate to the candidate's values, views on diversity, sense of teamwork, or other factors of importance to the organization. After it is developed, the script should be reviewed by a human resources expert to ensure it does not violate any civil rights or privacy rights laws. Once implemented, the script can be used to classify candidates quickly into categories, such as "exceeds requirements," "meets requirements," and "does not meet requirements." Those falling into the "does not meet requirements" category should politely be excused as quickly as possible.

In a rapidly moving market in which demand exceeds supply, delays in any aspect of the process will lead to the loss of well-qualified candidates. Each method of entry into the recruitment process should be scrutinized. An example of a script is provided in Figure 4.4.

The initial telephone interview is crucial to building rapport and selling the organization, assuming the candidate is a viable one. It also screens out any candidates who do not meet the needs of the job. If the candidate passes the telephone screening interview, schedule an in-person interview, let the department manager know of your progress, and ask him or her to also interview the candidate and conduct a tour. Be prepared for the candidate—if time allows, send

Figure 4.4: Phone Script for Screening Candidates

Hello, [name]. This is Robert Recruiter from Community General Hospital. I have received your resume for the night shift critical care position, and we are very interested in interviewing you. I would like to find out if you are still interested in the position and if so, would like to do a telephone interview as the first step. Would this be a convenient time? [If no, establish a time.]

First, I would like to ask you a few questions to help determine what you are looking for in a new position.

Conduct interview using questions tailored to your organization. Sample questions or items may include the following:

1. *Why are you seeking a new position at this time?*
2. *How long have you been employed in your current position?*
3. *What are you looking for in a new position?*
4. *What is your current salary? Does that include all differentials, overtime, and bonus payments?*
5. *Describe the environment in which you work best.*
6. *Describe your perfect day at work.*
7. *What is your shift preference?*
8. *What do you consider to be your strongest skill in nursing practice?*
9. *What is the most challenging situation you have faced?*

Let me tell you about our position and organization and what we seek in a candidate.

After the interview, thank the candidate. If he or she has passed the screening interview, set up an appointment for an in-person interview to take place within 48 hours, if possible.

information in advance related to the facility such as a brochure, the organization's benefits plans, and information about the department. Review your recruitment packet with a critical eye to ensure it is effective.

Candidates may not be ready to make a job change, or the department may not be the right fit at the time of the interview.

Figure 4.5: Handwritten Note to Prospective Candidate

Dear Lindsay,

I wanted to let you know of an exciting staff initiative that is underway on our unit. We have created a clinical excellence council, and the purpose of it is to advance clinical nursing practice in oncology. The staff developed new protocols for bone marrow transplant and also have had several exceptional lectures on innovative treatment options. A new clinical trial is also underway. The staff really want you as the oncology clinical nurse specialist, and we hope you will continue to consider working with us here on West Wing 7. Enclosed is a copy of our most recent newsletter.

Sincerely,

Brian Philip R.N., M.S.N.
Manager, West Wing 7

However, it is important to contact the candidate every few months. This keeps your facility at the top of the candidate's mind and assures him or her of your continued interest and attention.

Ensure Appropriate Tracking and Follow-through During the Process

Different procedures should be established to provide a tracking system for qualified candidates, depending on the level of candidate interest. For candidates who are well-qualified but are not ready to accept an offer at the present time, ensure as much as possible that they stay in the recruitment tracking queue:

- Call every few months and invite them to job fairs and open houses.
- Send information on any new programs.
- Send handwritten notes from the manager; these go a long way toward assuring the candidate he or she is regarded as a potentially valuable asset. Figure 4.5 provides an example of a such a note.

Tracking potential nursing candidates does not have to be elaborate. Use a tickler file (a reminder system in which you jot down what you need to do by date, and when that date arrives, you review its list of "to dos"; in this case, you would jot down the name and phone number of a candidate and file it for the date you want to follow up). Alternatively, use a spreadsheet to keep track of every candidate's position in the queue. In a rapidly moving market, you cannot afford to lose even one competent candidate.

Monitor and Evaluate Your Results

Part of a successful recruitment plan is to build in an evaluation process. Monitor your plan on a quarterly basis. To do this, review the plan and determine what results have occurred. If, for example, your open house was held, but not well attended, you can tweak or modify the communication plan. If your plan is not meeting strategic staffing needs, it must be revised.

Why monitor and evaluate? If your progress is not tracked and assessed, you cannot tell your success stories, nor can you know what areas or procedures to target if improvement is needed. Monitoring and evaluating help to identify sources that are effective, including those that are most and least cost effective. This process also evaluates the success of each recruiter and provides a communication mechanism on department effectiveness. Monitoring provides justification for the recruitment budget and helps to identify high turnover areas that can be a focus of improvement.

Performance Monitoring

A simple system to monitor each recruiter's success is to look at the number of contacts made each week, the number of interviews scheduled, and the number of resulting new hires. Targets can be set, and recruiters can be mentored and coached on the most effective ways to successfully recruit RNs.

When you are monitoring recruitment effectiveness, it is advisable to look at the actual positions that are recruited. One full-time equivalent (FTE) position may equal two part-time positions. Considering FTE levels alone can be misleading if you have a higher percentage of part-time staff. It is preferable to look at actual positions filled, not FTEs filled. Recruitment of part-time personnel takes as much time as that of full-time personnel. A department target should be established by month and by recruiter. When recruiters are not meeting their targets, they should be offered coaching, counseling, and additional job training. However, if a recruiter is not meeting hiring targets after assistance is offered, he or she should be replaced.

Monitoring by Source and Cost

A list of sources should be identified and number of hires and cost tracked monthly, quarterly, and at year end. Be sure you are using your money wisely.

Cost per hire is calculated on actual cost of the source that generated the leads (e.g., Internet, newspaper ad, refer-a-friend program) and does not include the recruiter's salary or departmental overhead. Figure 4.6 provides a template for monitoring by source and cost.

Figure 4.6: Monitoring by Source and Cost

Source	Hires	Cost/Hire
Refer-a-friend program	20	$200
Internet	16	$500
Job fairs	3	n/a
Schools of nursing	4	$20
Direct mail	12	$35
Walk-in applicants	4	n/a
Recruitment fairs	5	$500

Vacancy by Clinical Area

Vacancy rates by department will assist recruiters in identifying areas with historical recruitment problems and help nursing leadership intervene to evaluate the issues and determine resolutions. The vacancy by clinical area indicator looks at voluntary and involuntary position turnover by month and by quarter. Areas experiencing high turnover rates should be brought to the attention of nursing leadership, as they are costly in dollars, employee morale, and patient satisfaction.

Overall Cost per Hire

Overall cost per hire is usually obtained by dividing overall recruiter salaries and department expenses by the number of hires. The number is helpful for recruitment purposes, but may be viewed as artificially low, because none of the "backfill costs" of replacing vacant RN positions, such as agency staff, overtime, bonus payments, and orientation for new staff, are included. To obtain all recruitment costs, replacement costs should be factored into the equation.

Days to hire looks at the days from the time recruitment begins (date of request) to the actual hire. This statistic will identify the hard-to-fill areas in which different strategies are required. As an example, a critical care transplant RN vacancy may take 165 days to fill, and a postpartum RN vacancy may take 48 days to fill.

COMMUNICATION PLAN

Any great plan deserves an audience. Because of the current shortage of nurses, recruitment is an ongoing challenge; both the plan and results should be communicated on a regular basis. Monthly or quarterly management meetings, organizational intranet postings, newsletters, and board of directors meetings are a few forums in which the results should be reported. Statistical results of recruitment efforts should be provided to the manager to be communicated to the staff.

SUMMARY

This chapter should help you to develop an effective recruitment plan—one that clearly articulates goals and objectives and helps the organization evaluate its strengths, weaknesses, opportunities, and threats (a SWOT analysis).

Strategic workforce planning enables you to identify workforce needs by skill level category, department, shift, and any other critical characteristics. By targeting specific needs, recruitment strategies can be developed.

Developing a process for recruitment is important as a mechanism for guidance. A consistent process requires training, scripting, and monitoring the effectiveness of the recruitment personnel and processes. Sourcing strategies for obtaining candidates are identified, and suggestions for communicating the plan and results are provided.

The recruitment plan is now complete: you know your needs, you know how to meet your needs, you know how to search for candidates, you know how to budget, and you know how to develop key indicators and monitor your results. Chapter 5 will introduce you to the actual recruitment strategies that will build on the plan you have developed.

Strategies for Recruitment

INTRODUCTION

Clearly planned strategies for long- and short-term recruitment will help ensure that your nurse staffing needs are met. This chapter presents a number of strategies, along with ways that these strategies can be implemented. Targeting the right employees requires an understanding of what is important to them. Tips are suggested to meet the differing needs of the RN candidates you want to work at your facility.

In addition, the characteristics of generation X and Net generation employees are described, as their needs and desires differ from preceding generations. Understanding them will ensure recruitment and retention of this vital resource in your nursing arena.

Long-term recruitment from grade school through high school is necessary to get students interested and exposed to a career in nursing. Methods to grow your own RNs via local high schools are described. Finally, effective nursing student strategies are identified, as ongoing success in recruitment and retention within this population will ensure that your patient care needs are met year after year.

In the previous chapter, a number of planning strategies were identified. Now is the time to implement your plan. Following the market is often ineffective—leading the market is very effective. This chapter will present ways to lead the market and provide many practical ideas that can be implemented for the short and long term.

ANTICIPATE NEEDS OF TOMORROW'S EMPLOYEES

Understanding future trends is very important to your recruitment strategy. No one strategy will work, because different segments of the workforce have different needs. Therefore, many different options for recruitment must be available. The following sections predict the needs of various types of future nursing employees and discuss particular strategies that will be effective for recruiting each segment.

Future Employees Will Want More Personal Time in Lieu of Additional Compensation

Throughout the United States, people are seeking to balance work time and leisure time. Many employees prefer time over money—increased personal time is more important to them than a higher salary. More employees are opting for more leisure time, and work-life balance is increasingly important (Neuhauser 2002).

An example of effective recruitment strategies that respond to this trend include offering part-time, weekend-only, and 12-hour-shift programs. These allow employees to consolidate their work week and devote blocks of time to meeting their lifestyle needs.

Future Employees Will Seek to Balance Work and Family Life

Rather than see life as an "either/or" proposition, requiring a choice of either a satisfying work or family life, a trend toward effectively balancing these two aspects of life has emerged. Employees are seeking time for family obligations and time-saving amenities.

Effective recruitment will highlight the opportunity to balance work and family in a particular position. Potential recruitment strategies include offering on-site child care, providing resource and referral services for child care and elder care, and offering "convenience" services such as dry cleaning pick-up, take-out meals, and on-site shopping opportunities like book fairs, jewelry sales, glove sales, and toy sales.

A Subgroup of Future Employees Will Want to Carry the Greatest Workload

Rather than the balance described above, a subgroup may wish to work additional hours and earn additional compensation. In each generation of staff, this population exists and adds great value to the organization because of its willingness to work additional hours.

Recruitment of this type of worker involves promoting bonus-hour opportunities, offering occasional-staffing options, and identifying areas where opportunities for additional hours are always available. Limiting overtime or bonus opportunities for this population is a sure way to create turnover.

Future Employees Will Be Looking for Employers that Offer a Stable and Secure Environment, Especially Related to Pay, Hours, and Benefits

Nurses of the future will be well aware of trends in healthcare, particularly downsizing, mergers, and acquisitions. Although they may not expect to spend their entire career at one location, as some nurses did in the past, they do expect a basic level of security.

Recruitment techniques that will work for this type of employee include highlighting your track record in this area, emphasizing your no-layoff policy, and profiling the benefits you offer, such as health insurance, disability, long-term care, life insurance, and paid time off.

Future Employees Will Seek Professional Growth and Promotional Opportunities

Employees may have a clear career path in mind that includes promotion from staff nurse to various other positions, including staff support and managerial roles. For example, a nurse may seek both additional education and additional responsibilities in the work place.

Recruiting this type of nurse calls for showcasing career pathways, promotional ladders, and transfer policies. Statistics on promotions from within may be cited. Real-life stories or testimonials of nurses who have climbed the career ladder at your institution may be used. Recruitment should also highlight education benefits, including on-site in-service training and conferences, external conferences and conventions, and tuition reimbursement for college courses.

Future Employees Will Seek Opportunities to Be Creative and Work in Self-directed Teams

Today's classroom is moving away from hierarchy to collaborative education. Tomorrow's employees will want less bureaucracy and more ability to develop collaborative and self-directed solutions to work challenges.

Effective recruitment will showcase your participative decision-making model and the high-profile role of staff nurses. Highlight the accomplishments of staff nurses and use your staff to recruit the populations commonly known as generation X and the Net generation by taking staff members to job fairs, career days, and school recruitment programs. Showcasing your web-based education, use of technology, and interactive computer-based education capabilities will attract this group of employees.

GENERATION X ENTREPRENEURS AND NET GENERATION EMPLOYEES

In addition to understanding future employee trends, you will need to understand that the new generations of employees you will recruit and retain in your facility were raised in a different social context and have different attitudes about work and employment. The successful organization will develop different strategies over the long term to attract this new worker; the first step is to understand the differences in the Net and X generations.

Generation X Employees

Generation X employees were born between 1965 and 1977 and are often described as cynical, pessimistic, and reluctant to make commitments. Currently in their 20s and 30s, generation X employees want greater autonomy and less bureaucracy. They are loyal to work and not employer, and they change jobs frequently if their demands are not met. They are choosing freelance or agency employment over alignment with an organization. This is seen in the number of RNs who are choosing to work in a nursing agency at a high rate of pay. Top-down control management is undesirable; teamwork and creativity are desired.

Employment Considerations

An awareness of the characteristics given above enables employers to know how to target this group of recruits. Unleashing their talent and ideas and addressing hospital image stereotypes are positive efforts for the profession and can only be good for future nurses.

Many nurse leaders and recruiters want to understand more about how to recruit and retain generation X nurses. First, recruitment should focus on the desires of generation X employees. This employee population is well-suited for areas in which challenge and career growth can be found, such as critical care settings and cross-training opportunities between similar units. They thrive in a unit culture that is open to innovation and change, with a participative manager who is accepting of employee input. Service orientation should be stressed and opportunities for service identified, such as charity clinics, disadvantaged population services, and community outreach services.

The employer also needs to understand the importance of free time to this generation of employees and their unwillingness to work too many additional hours, reflecting their need for work-life balance. This key employee group should be sold on the generous vacation allowance nursing offers, the opportunity for working with diverse groups of staff and patients, the flexibility you can offer in career growth, and your site's continuous learning opportunities. Having other generation X nurses assist in the recruitment process and answer questions, as well as present what attracted them to your facility, is very beneficial.

Net Generation Employees

In contrast, Net generation members were born between 1980 and 1999 and are very different from their predecessor generation. This generation is open to and actively seeks the helping professions, desires job stability, and wants to work in organizations.

Technical competency in leaders is valued. Net generation employees have been exposed to technology for most of their lives, view it as an essential part of any job, and find it empowering. This is the first generation that is more skilled than adults in technology.

Various descriptions of the Net generation have been offered. Generally, the group is viewed as serious and sophisticated about life. Members of this generation tend to be assertive, with high self-esteem and self-confidence. They are oriented toward teams and achievement and have a strong sense of civic duty and social ethic.

These characteristics make the Net generation of RNs very valuable to the institution. To recruit them, your organization must demonstrate the following:

- a commitment to social responsibility in the community
- a continuous learning environment
- a focus on excellence in all aspects of organizational life

In addition, the opportunity for teamwork and shared leadership must be provided.

When recruiting this age group, profiling how you can meet the needs in their lives is beneficial. As an example, you can have a team-oriented interviewing process at the clinical unit in which they interact with various staff members from that unit. You can provide a demonstration of how the organization uses technology and the Internet for patient care delivery, communication, scheduling, staffing, and so forth.

Build on their interests by showcasing opportunities for community outreach and involvement and providing a calendar of continuing education opportunities, especially those that are available through technology such as CD-ROM or the Internet.

LONG-TERM RECRUITMENT

In addition to understanding the generational differences in those you will be recruiting, it is also necessary to consider many different long-term strategies for recruitment. It is never too early to introduce nursing as a career option, even at the elementary school level, and exposure should be continued throughout the educational process. Other recruitment endeavors that occur over time include targeting nursing school students prior to graduation and building relationships over time. Re-entry RNs can make a strong contribution to your organization if you are willing to make the commitment needed to bring this group back into the workforce.

Grade School (Kindergarten Through Sixth Grade)

Educators state that children decide by the fifth grade which careers are desirable and undesirable. Few formal opportunities exist for introducing nursing as a career choice for this age group. However, creative recruiters can employ any or all of the following tactics:

- Contact schools in your community and offer the services of your recruiters or nursing representatives.
- Contact youth groups, such as church groups, the YMCA, Girl Scouts, and Boy Scouts, and offer to talk about nursing as a career.
- Present nursing as a positive career choice when parents and area businesses are invited to classrooms to discuss what they do.
- Purchase or create coloring books or activity books that highlight the diverse work of nurses and distribute them at the elementary schools in your area.

For this age group, the presentation should be easy to understand and geared toward introducing the idea of nursing as a career to young people of both genders. Hands-on experiences are always appreciated by grade school students and can be simply accomplished with sessions using a few tools such as a thermometer, a watch, a stethoscope, and a blood pressure cuff.

Junior High/Middle School and High School Students (Seventh Through Twelfth Grade)

Targeting students at the junior high and high school levels presents additional options because of the increased age, attention span, and interests of the youths. The tactics discussed in the following sections do not require much time and are important for your long-term needs. Assign a recruiter to be responsible for the school-age population. Results will not be immediately apparent, but the efforts will be very worthwhile, as teens in your community choose nursing because of the exposure to nursing as a career choice.

General Strategies for Attracting Teens to a Nursing Career

Several general strategies can be used to highlight nursing as a career in the teen population. For example, your facility might sponsor contests with a nursing theme and age-appropriate prizes. You might also work with school libraries to purchase age-appropriate books on nursing or provide the libraries with donated books.

Using MTV-like videos that "sell" nursing is an especially effective tactic, because this type of presentation medium is so pervasive in their social context. Once advertised through career counselors, with program fliers, in local newspapers, or by direct mail, these can be inexpensively broadcast on local cable television or shown during career fairs at schools. The National Student Nurses Association has prepared a video, "Nursing: The Ultimate Adventure," targeted to high school students. The American Nurses Association has joined Sigma Theta Tau, the honor society for nursing, and other nursing and healthcare organizations to develop a media campaign. At the time of this writing, Johnson & Johnson is engaged in a major campaign to increase nurse recruitment; more suggestions are provided in an excellent listing of online resources available in the Johnson & Johnson brochure and included on their web site (Figure 5.1). These are beneficial recruitment tools and are recommended as part of your recruitment tool kit for your outreach activities.

For more creative ways of exposing teens to nursing, think about where teens congregate—their school, community centers, shopping malls, movies, and restaurants. Talk to local merchants about inexpensive ways to reach teens. A booth with age-appropriate in-

Figure 5.1: Choosing a Career in Nursing—Online Resources

www.discovernursing.com
Johnson & Johnson Campaign for Nursing's Future

www.nln.org
National League for Nursing

www.nursesource.org
Nurses for a Healthier Tomorrow

www.nsna.org
National Student Nurses' Association

www.ana.org
American Nurses Association

www.nursingsociety.org
Honor Society of Nursing/Sigma Theta Tau International

www.aone.org
American Organization of Nurse Executives

www.aacn.nche.edu
American Association of Colleges of Nursing

Source: Johnson & Johnson Health Care Systems, Inc. 2002. "Because I Am a Nurse." The Campaign for Nursing's Future.

formation on health and free giveaways is one option. A food court may also be an ideal place to reach teens.

Reaching Teens Through Schools

An easy way to connect with teens is through their schools. The best way to start developing school relationships is by contacting school guidance counselors or administrative personnel. Developing ongoing relationships with the guidance counselors is invaluable in promoting nursing as a career choice. You should meet with the guidance counselors or administrators at least twice a year. Invite them to a breakfast at a local restaurant or at your facility. Share healthcare career opportunities with them, emphasizing nursing in particular. Provide information on educational requirements, financial assistance, student job opportunities, web site addresses for students to access, and career opportunities.

In addition to interacting with school staff, it is essential to interact directly with students. Provide presentations during career days, either at the school or at your institution. This usually involves an hour-long discussion in which a presentation is made on the RN role, educational requirements, salary, job responsibilities, and career mobility. Holding your own career nights with booths developed and staffed by your nurses and other healthcare professionals is also an effective way to reach students. Hold these in local school gyms or cafeterias and invite students and parents. Provide information and giveaways, such as mouse pads, key chains, Post-It® pads, tiny radios, or similar items printed with a nursing theme.

Sponsoring a "Future Nurses Club," offering an RN-shadowing program, or conducting a nursing camp will help reach teens in high school:

- The Future Nurses Club may be scheduled to meet monthly and may include tours, discussion groups, "RN stories" from staff, education, videos, book discussions, and demonstrations.
- Shadowing programs are designed to allow students to follow an RN for several hours. Shadowing experiences must be carefully selected, as the wrong opportunity can frighten students away from the RN role.
- A week-long summer nursing camp can be offered to high school juniors and seniors. Such a camp promotes nursing as a career while offering an experiential program. The camp may include a shadowing program, cardiopulmonary resuscitation (CPR) classes, RN testimonials, tours of selected hospital units, field trips, first-aid classes, coursework discussion groups, web-based exposure to healthcare sites, web-based or CD-ROM education, and summer employment opportunities.

One of the most valuable recruitment tools is the development of a nursing career "grow your own" program. This is a partnership between a local high school and your human resources and nursing education departments. The program begins prior to the senior year, and 12 to 15 students are selected. Steps are outlined in Figure 5.2. This type of program provides an ideal way for families with limited resources to afford college tuition and allows students to develop a long-term career in your organization.

If your organization does not have available resources for student support, other options are scholarships and loan forgiveness. Often, philanthropic organizations can assist in this endeavor, and a number of grant opportunities also exist, especially for disadvantaged students, through foundations, the federal government, and local organizations.

This strategy requires a significant commitment by the organization, but it pays big dividends. Be sure to structure agreements for this type of program to years of service in return for being a part of this career development strategy.

Loans and loan forgiveness programs, along with scholarship programs, are effective ways to recruit teens who want a career in nursing. If you have planned for these and can fund them, they will assist you in your ability to attract bright, service-oriented teens to the profession. They also may provide for those who could not otherwise afford nursing school the opportunity to attend, with a payback to the facility in terms of years of service.

Understanding Teen Expectations

When you are reaching out to this audience, it is important to understand that teenagers are not miniature adults. They have certain expectations that must be met to attract them to the nursing profession. The expectations are listed below, along with some ways to

Figure 5.2: A Grow-Your-Own Program for Students

Time Frame	Path	Enablers
Junior year, high school	Students apply and are selected for healthcare track	Partnership with high school, human resources, and nursing; small class size (maximum 12)
Senior year, high school	Hospital education department provides assistance in education and training for students to be trained as RN-assistive personnel	Curriculum designed by educational specialists and nurse educators; skills labs provided; instructors provided
High school graduation, age 18	Graduates apply for RN-assistive personnel positions; full- or part-time are selected	Open positions made available; supportive and timely human resources process
Post–high school graduation	Students work full- or part-time with full tuition reimbursement for pursuit of nursing degree at local school	Tuition reimbursement; flexible schedule; supportive manager; assigned career coach
Two to four years post–high school graduation	Students graduate from nursing program and become full-time RNS	Publicity; open positions for new graduates; ongoing training and career development

meet the expectations when presenting career options in nursing to this group.

Teens want to be involved in a career that features autonomy and independence, critical thinking, and continuous learning. These may be addressed by:

- identifying the ongoing critical thinking and decision making inherent in nursing;
- identifying the importance of doing well academically to meet entry standards and successfully complete the curriculum;
- discussing the importance of science and math and how the content is used every day in the nursing profession;
- stressing the autonomous nature of the RN job and the moment-to-moment decision making that occurs; and
- providing concrete examples or case studies about decisions RNs make, often in life-or-death situations.

Teens want variety, challenge, and career choices in their work life future. To highlight opportunities in nursing, consider:

- discussing the many settings in which a career in nursing can be applied and providing concrete examples on how, what, when, and where nursing is practiced;
- identifying career mobility, career change opportunities, and the ability to work both in the United States and abroad;.
- describing how, as interests and needs change, many career transitions are possible within nursing; and
- profiling the many career opportunities and pathways that nursing provides, such as specialty RNs in emergency departments, critical care, and pediatrics; and advanced practice nurses, including nurse practitioner, nurse anesthetist, and clinical nurse specialist; as well as other nurse options such as administration, education, research, and consultation.

Teens want to know that career advancement and leadership opportunities are available. This need may be addressed by:

- stressing the many opportunities that are possible for nurses who seek leadership careers and providing examples from your institution;

- identifying the opportunity for RNs with advanced education to become managers, directors, vice presidents, chief operating officers, and chief executive officers; and
- identifying the many career advancement options in health-care, education, industry, and consultation.

Teens want to make an impact. They want to improve society through a "make a difference" career that involves collaboration. To highlight opportunities in nursing, consider:

- stressing the difference a nurse makes on a daily basis in the lives of patients and families and providing examples;
- demonstrating the impact nurses have had locally, regionally, nationally, and internationally in terms of improving health and saving lives;
- treating the topics of illness, suffering, death, treatments, and blood with great sensitivity, if they arise (teens may be fearful of illness and thus avoid nursing unless this is handled sensitively); and
- providing information on the collaborative nature of the profession and identifying the many opportunities for collaboration with physicians, pharmacists, social workers, clergy, nutritionists, and other healthcare professionals.

Teens want to be sure their chosen profession will support them financially and will be worth the initial investment for education, especially if the family has limited resources. You may address this concern by:

- stressing the availability of nursing school loan programs, loan forgiveness programs, tuition assistance, and scholarships;
- providing the salary ranges for a variety of jobs within nursing;
- identifying nursing as a stable career choice with many options for the future; and

- conducting presentations for parents about nursing school funding options.

Teens who are service oriented and want to help others and make a difference will be attracted to the profession of nursing. Nursing as a career must be presented carefully, with planned experiences and discussions provided as the teens mature.

Nursing Students

An effective long-term strategy for recruitment is building relationships with nursing students. These individuals have selected nursing as a career and need to understand why they should select your institution for their practice setting. Interacting with nursing students early in the education process will pay big dividends. A number of strategies are outlined below.

Leverage faculty to help with recruitment. Offer summer and other employment to faculty from schools of nursing. Hold continuing education events in partnership with them. Assign a hospital manager or education "buddy" while faculty are conducting clinical student rotations to ensure high-quality student experiences.

Offer many nursing student clinical rotations in your facility, and ensure the student has an excellent clinical experience. Follow up with each student via mailings, continuing education, social offerings, and telephone contact.

Hire nursing students between their junior and senior year for summer unlicensed assistive personnel or patient companion work. Provide education, mentoring, and support. Allow them to work part-time and over holiday periods. Stay in touch throughout their senior year and offer positions after graduation.

Hold social events during students' junior and senior years. Take staff nurses with you who are graduates of the targeted school to answer questions and discuss positions at wine and cheese parties (be sure your attendees are of legal age to drink alcohol), luncheons, theme parties, outdoor concerts with dinner under a tent, picnics, or an event at a venue in your community that would appeal to students.

Hold a resume-writing and interviewing course for nursing students. Use role-play to showcase your interviewing and selection techniques. This also teaches valuable skills to the student.

Offer nursing internships or extended orientation for new graduates. Use these programs as a recruitment tool. Emphasize the sheltered environment, ongoing continuing education, web-based individualized learning, and the availability of a consistent preceptor.

Hold a successful nursing student open house. RN student open houses are inexpensive and easy to implement and produce results. Figure 5.3 provides guidelines to ensure success. A successful open house is one from which several new hires result.

Re-entry RNs

Reaching out to registered nurses who are out of active practice is another recruitment strategy. The re-entry RN may require an extended orientation or a re-entry course. Community colleges may offer a re-entry course, or the healthcare facility may develop a course on its own or in partnership with other healthcare agencies or organizations. Demand for a re-entry program should be assessed prior to embarking on program development; if no more than five RNs are interested in attending, it may not be worthwhile. A re-entry program must also take into consideration the gap in practice and what the majority of re-entry RNs will need in terms of coursework, clinical setting, and mentoring.

Re-entry programs are a long-term strategy, considering the investment that is required, whether your facility offers the course or it is outsourced. They require a facility, instructors, clinical rotations,

Figure 5.3: Guidelines for a Successful RN Student Open House

What you need: Clinical managers with enthusiasm, space for the event, recruiters, refreshments, recruitment materials

- Open house for student RNs is scheduled quarterly or biannually during the senior year, and all clinical managers are notified of dates for the year, so they can be present to "sell" their unit.
- All department profiles that describe the unit, type of patient, staffing ratios, nursing delivery model, philosophy, etc., are evaluated and updated to reflect positive attributes and are placed in an attractive folder, along with hospital and nursing information.
- Mailing lists for the targeted schools of nursing are obtained from the state nursing association.
- Ad copy for the event is written and provided to local schools of nursing, targeting student nursing publications, and copy is prepared for direct-mail two weeks prior to event. Door prizes are obtained, such as key chains, Post-It® notes, refrigerator magnets.
- Refreshments are ordered, recruitment packets are prepared, and all details are checked to ensure completeness one week prior to event.
- Clinical managers and recruiters prepare for event two hours in advance, setting up booths, preparing marketing materials, and ensuring all departmental representatives are present.
- Each attendee signs in; the names and addresses will be used for door prizes and future recruitment endeavors.
- Managers and recruiters screen, interview, and make offers to candidates contingent on their passing pre-employment require-ments, with the understanding that the student must pass state licensing exams to function as an RN. A start date is established.
- Job fair hire rates are tracked and follow-up is completed.
- Recruiters evaluate job fair and identify ways to improve for the next quarter.

a classroom, and skills lab training. Implement this strategy if you have many open positions and positions that are in general areas. Be sure re-entry RNs commit to working full- or part-time after com-pletion. "Letters of commitment" should be signed prior to embark-ing on this strategy to offset the cost of the program.

SHORT-TERM FINANCIAL STRATEGIES

A strong compensation system is required and may need to be enhanced by short-term incentive programs to recruit staff. Given the immediate need to fill critical areas, short-term strategies are an important part of recruitment. These strategies often include and even require fiscal incentives, especially in markets with severe RN shortages.

Compensation

An effective compensation strategy is a baseline recruitment tool. RNs will be swayed by the best starting wage for a new graduate or a higher hourly rate than they are currently making. Often, organizations are penny-wise and pound-foolish. To recruit effectively, you must offer a competitive market wage with ranges of pay that are frequently adjusted. If you are not competitive in the market, address this first. Financial incentives for recruiting new staff will be ineffective if your base wages are too low.

Should salary compression become an internal issue, it must be addressed as part of retention. Compression occurs when you are hiring external staff, be it new graduates or experienced RNs, at a higher wage than that earned by internal staff. Although this may result in the successful recruitment of staff, it will have a negative impact on retention of your internal staff and is short-sighted.

An August 2001 Florida Hospital Association study on recruitment and retention, "Finding and Keeping Nurses: What Is Working?," provides insight into financial incentives that hospitals are using to recruit RNs. Results are presented in Figure 5.4.

While getting RNs in the door requires a competitive base wage, RNs usually also inquire about benefits, with an emphasis on vacation, health insurance, pay raises, and shift differentials. You can stay ahead of the recruiting game by being the first in the market to offer innovative incentives or benefits not offered by competitors. Be sure

Figure 5.4: Financial Incentives Used by Hospitals to Recruit Nurses

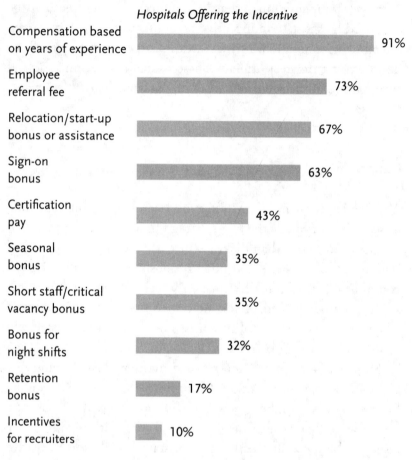

Hospitals Offering the Incentive

Compensation based on years of experience — 91%

Employee referral fee — 73%

Relocation/start-up bonus or assistance — 67%

Sign-on bonus — 63%

Certification pay — 43%

Seasonal bonus — 35%

Short staff/critical vacancy bonus — 35%

Bonus for night shifts — 32%

Retention bonus — 17%

Incentives for recruiters — 10%

Source: Adapted from Florida Hospital Association (2001). Used with permission.

to assess the affordability of such incentives and choose the areas in which they will apply. Benefits that may attract RNs include paid time off, on-site child care, cafeteria benefit plans, and flexible staffing options such as part-time, alternative shifts, and compressed work weeks.

A recent review of classified ads in newspapers and nursing publications demonstrates the variety of incentives being offered to attract RNs, some of which you may want to consider:

- Work 24 hours on the weekend and receive 40 hours pay.
- Receive a night-shift differential of $5 to $10 per hour.
- Commit to 72 hours per month and receive $35 per hour.
- Receive a $10,000 sign-on bonus for critical care RNs.
- Weekender program—receive $10 per hour shift differential on days and $20 on nights.
- In-house registry—receive up to $40 per hour.
- Receive new graduate RN hire-on bonus of $2,500.
- Work three 12-hour shifts for full-time pay and benefits.

Although these are not applicable to all areas because of affordability issues, they can be used in areas with recruitment challenges. Review agency overtime and internal bonus costs and use new incentives to recruit staff and reduce premium rate pay. When implementing these programs, it is wise to offer them to internal staff first. It is also prudent to develop guidelines for the programs that enable the facility to terminate the program with 30 days notice or change the rate of pay. In today's economic environment, the programs may have a short life because of fiscal considerations and the changing market. Staff in each of the incentive programs should sign a copy of the guidelines, which should be placed in their personnel file upon hire.

Other Programs

A few of the most effective short-term financial strategies that will enable you to recruit in your market for hard-to-fill areas are defined in the list below.

Before implementing these recruitment strategies, it is important for you to consider and analyze several variables. How affordable is the strategy? How will it be paid for? What is the anticipated duration of the strategy? How will the strategy affect internal staff, both positively and negatively? Only after these questions are answered should the strategy be implemented.

- *Weekender program.* In this program, a high weekend shift differential is offered to .6 FTE for working all weekends for a three- to six-month period.
- *Compressed work week.* Nurses work three 12-hour shifts for full-time benefits and 36 hours compensation.
- *Night life program.* In this program, a high shift differential is offered for working nights for three to six consecutive months.
- *Hire-on bonuses in areas of short supply.* In this program, areas of short supply, such as critical care units and operating rooms, offer hire-on bonuses. Bonuses may vary from $1,000 to $3,000 or more. Half should be paid upon hire, and half should be paid in six months.
- *Refer-a-friend program.* Refer-a-friend efforts are very cost-effective programs that you can start and stop at any time. Such a program should be included in any effective recruitment program. Provide a financial incentive or a perk such as a parking spot or gift certificates to employees who refer others to your facility. You can offer a grand prize such as a large cash prize or a trip to the staff member who recruits the most people.

  An ideal time for refer-a-friend programs is when a new staff member mentions an issue at his or her previous place of employment that is causing staff to seek new opportunities. One hospital filled all of its open ER positions by using this tactic, and the referring friend won a large cash prize. The recruited employees were thrilled with their new positions; thus, everyone felt they had come out ahead.

STRATEGIES THAT SET YOU APART

Many recruitment strategies have been mentioned in this chapter. The key to success for recruitment is to differentiate your institution in your market. How?

- Network with others about recruitment ideas.
- Look at what the competition is doing.
- Search web sites and national journals for ideas.
- Use a recruitment task force to brainstorm.
- Review the literature.
- Attend local and national conferences.

You can differentiate yourself through compensation, benefits, and professional nursing practice. Many of these have already been discussed, but they bear repeating Other categories can also be considered, such as reputation, culture, and organizational strengths. Choose the ones in which you excel and develop ways of creating a competitive advantage.

Compensation

- Wages ahead of the market
- Higher shift differentials
- Incentive programs, for example, weekend and night life incentives
- Hire-on bonuses
- Higher-than-market raises or frequent internal raises
- Career path with higher-than-market increases between levels
- Extra-shift bonuses
- Double pay for overtime in crisis periods
- Critical care or specialty differentials

Benefits

- On-site child care
- On-site sick child care
- Convenience services (e.g., dry cleaning pick-up, take-out meals, cash machine on site)

- Health and wellness services (e.g., classes, counseling, fitness center, weight control programs)
- Alternative work schedules (e.g., part-time, job sharing, compressed work week, flexible scheduling)
- Tuition reimbursement, scholarships, loan forgiveness
- Adoption assistance
- Matched savings
- Paid time off in excess of competitors
- Resource and referral services
- Tax-free savings accounts for dependent care and medical expenses
- Employee assistance programs
- Emergency employee loans

Professional Nursing Practices and Support

- Magnet Nursing Services Recognition Program for Excellence (American Nurses Credentialing Center)
- Participative decision-making model
- Career growth through established career paths
- Nursing excellence award mentoring
- RN to BSN to MSN tracks geared to adult worker
- "Earn while you learn" continuing web-based education
- Renewal opportunities for stress education offered on site
- Short sabbaticals with pay that focus on enhancement of an aspect of nursing practice or patient care delivery
- Recognition for preceptors

Use the unique attributes of your organization to recruit into your facility. Remember—first impressions count! Make sure each interaction with potential recruits is very positive in word and deed. Your materials must differentiate you. Your staff must differentiate you. Your application process must differentiate you. Your interactions must differentiate you.

Finally, differentiate yourself in follow-up. Send a note to or call the candidate after the interview. If he or she accepts the job, set the tone by having a letter of welcome sent from the hiring manager or chief nurse executive. A small floral arrangement can be sent to new managers and to staff, if the budget allows.

SUMMARY

Strategies for recruitment are both long and short term, and you must address both to be effective. Individualizing your strategies to target populations—new graduates versus re-entry RNs, as an example, will ensure success. You can use various methods to recruit RNs, from innovative benefit packages to flexible staffing options such as weekend positions and compressed work weeks. Borrow ideas from other industries and network to identify other creative ideas for recruiting RNs. Keep your eye on the competition, but do not copy your competitors. Instead, do it better.

This chapter presented many recruitment ideas that should be tailored to your particular situation. Determine what will fit within your budget and what will work best for you. Do only what you are sure you can deliver. Always try to be the first in your market to offer unique programs.

This section concludes with Appendix 5.1, "Toolbox: 100 Ways to Recruit RNs." This can serve as a checklist to see how you are doing or be used to develop new ideas. Items are listed by category.

REFERENCES

Florida Hospital Association. 2001. "FHA Eye on the Health Care Worker. Florida's Nursing Shortage: It's Here and It Is Getting Worse." [Online article; retrieved Feb. 25, 2002.] Tallahassee, FL: Florida Hospital Association. www.fha.org /allproducts/html.

Neuhauser, P.C. 2002. "Building a High-retention Culture in Healthcare: Fifteen Ways to Get Good People to Stay." *Journal of Nursing Administration* 32 (9): 470–78.

Image/Public Relations

1. Profile in the local newspaper a compelling patient care story in which an RN played a major role.
2. Develop a shadowing program for high school students.
3. Promote nursing as a career that is highly versatile—engage staff in school job fairs.
4. Hold an "invitation only" event with a celebrity or athlete to pitch your healthcare facility.
5. Stage e-mail postcard campaigns that may yield results of 5 to 15 percent.
6. Purchase radio, cinema, and cable television advertising.
7. Use transit advertising (billboards) in heavy traffic areas.
8. "Adopt" a middle school or junior high school and introduce nursing as a career through presentations, displays, literature selections, career days, clubs, and interactions with school personnel.
9. Develop multimedia advertising campaigns.
10. Advertise in publications that will be distributed at large trade shows.
11. Advertise in specialty-based nursing journals, newsletters, and other publications.
12. Provide RNs to speak at community events, bookstores, service-oriented clubs, etc., to promote nursing and to recruit.
13. Obtain and promote magnet hospital status.
14. Hold a "Top 10" contest to develop lists indicating why RNs choose to work at your facility; use it in recruitment ads.
15. Use "hot jobs" listings on cafeteria tents, posting boards, intranet, and internal publications that target hard-to-fill areas.
16. Advertise in local newspapers, community centers, churches, and community-based organizations.

17. Use an internal newsletter for "hot jobs" that lists job openings and incentives or bonuses being offered for target jobs.
18. Have a recruitment booth and materials at all hospital events for community education, continuing education, seminars, etc.

Compensation and Benefits

19. Offer a refer-a-friend bonus to existing staff. Assign a higher bonus for hard-to-fill areas. Example: $500 for medical/surgical and $1,000 to $3,000 for critical care.
20. Offer loan forgiveness programs to graduating students based on years of service.
21. Offer nursing scholarships in return for work commitment.
22. Offer cafeteria-style benefits to meet the individualized needs of today's RNs.
23. Offer hiring bonus in difficult-to-fill areas.
24. Pay premium rates to recruit the cross-trained RN who can work in any area within a section (medical/surgical, adult critical care, pediatrics, etc.).
25. Grow your own RNs—provide tuition assistance to entry-level workers for nursing school.
26. Offer tuition reimbursement as a recruitment incentive.
27. Offer a transportation option or subsidy.
28. Provide child care on site or near site, or offer a referral service.
29. Offer the highest wages in the market—then watch as competitors match it.
30. Create your own internal resource agency that matches agency rates and ensure staff are multiskilled.
31. Offer spousal or significant-other benefits that include assistance in finding jobs, job relocation, and support services.
32. Offer paid continuing education days on or off site.
33. Offer incentives to recruiters for hiring qualified candidates.

34. Offer incentive-based pay or bonus payments in target areas that recognize higher-level competencies.
35. Offer a weekender program with a high differential of $10 to $20 per hour.
36. Offer premiums for "hot skills."
37. Offer a "hire onto full-time" bonus for part-time personnel.
38. Offer "bridging" of benefits—if an employee returns within six months of resigning, all benefits stay intact.

Staffing and Scheduling

39. Use a "resource pool" strategy to employ non-benefits-eligible RNs. Encourage them to move into full-time and part-time positions and float within clinical sections; provide a differential.
40. Offer flexible staffing options—4 hour, 8 hour, or 12 hour shifts, weekender, night life, etc.
41. Offer part-time, full-time, and PRN positions.
42. Guarantee hours—no low-census time.
43. Hire RNs into a temporary assistance pool, even if no positions are available. After three months, place them in a float position or on a clinical unit.
44. Use traveler RNs to fill gaps and then recruit the most qualified.
45. Offer three 12-hour shifts for full-time benefits.
46. Provide nine-month positions in areas where census declines in the summer.
47. Offer seven days on/seven days off as a recruitment strategy.

Student Recruitment

48. Develop a work/study program for high school students.
49. Hold a nursing camp for junior high/middle school or early

high school students for a week each summer. Offer first-aid, shadowing, RN testimonials, work opportunities, healthcare-related field trips, CPR, and web instruction.

50. Reach out to junior high students using the National Student Nurses' Association's MTV-style video.
51. Offer summer externships to nursing students.
52. Offer "how to interview" classes for student RNs—this builds rapport and skills.
53. Offer nursing faculty summer opportunities for employment.
54. Hold biannual events for nursing faculty to build relationships and provide ongoing continuing education.
55. Recruit high school seniors into entry-level nursing positions and offer tuition assistance for RN courses leading to a degree.
56. Sell new graduates on the high-tech aspects of your organization and demonstrate how you are superior.
57. Offer a new graduate internship.
58. Offer an individualized career path that starts in high school—map the RN career for the student.

Professional Growth and Development

59. Guarantee each new employee an experienced preceptor.
60. Provide a career pathway for each prospective RN to demonstrate career advancement in the organization.
61. Grow your own specialty nurses by choosing your best and brightest general staff RNs and provide skills and training with an assigned mentor.
62. Retrain those RNs who are in areas that are being downsized into a new career path.
63. Tap the 45- to 50-year-old RN who has been out of the workforce, and provide a career re-entry course.

64. Highlight nursing involvement in committees, task forces, governance, management, and clinical practice to showcase the nursing voice in decision making.

General Strategies

65. Hold an open house for RNs every quarter. Have managers from clinical units profile their unit with a booth or display and do screening and interviewing, and make job offers on the spot.
66. Hold an electronic recruitment fair in which a select group of managers review web-based resumes; expedite the process for job interviews and selections.
67. Call every qualified RN in good standing who has left in the last year and ask them to return. Offer competitive compensation and benefits packages. Offer a rehire bonus in hard-to-fill areas.
68. Leave cards at your hairdresser and ask for recruitment assistance.
69. Have specialty unit staff write a personal letter about his or her unit and send it to target specialty RNs in the area via direct mail.
70. Promote the continuing education courses you offer.
71. Use your own web site, as well as commercial sites, to recruit.
72. Attend target nursing job fairs in the area.
73. Explore international recruitment and understand the requirements and regulations surrounding it.
74. Choose creative staff RNs to be on an RN recruitment committee and empower them to develop strategies.
75. Choose an industry outside of healthcare and borrow one good recruitment idea.
76. Aggressively recruit agency and PRN personnel by determining what they need to become staff members.

77. Initiate a 48-hour interview-selection timeline.
78. Ask new hires who the best RNs were at their last place of employment and call them about positions, or ask the referring RN to do so.
79. Involve staff in filling openings on their unit, using word of mouth.
80. Work with a minority recruitment firm to enhance cultural diversity in your healthcare facility.
81. Hold focus groups to identify why RNs chose your facility.
82. Tap your volunteer pool and recruit from these into support positions for nursing. Hold a job fair for older workers and ensure positions are geared to them.
83. Offer external clinical specialty continuing education days, with continuing education units (CEU), and offer recruitment services at the event. Capture demographic data on attendees for follow-up.
84. Place employment kiosks in your healthcare organization and local businesses and community centers.
85. Take advantage of top-performing healthcare recruitment web sites.
86. Use employee referral programs online and relaunch with a new name and incentives every nine months.
87. Promote "nurse enablers" as a recruitment strategy. Focus on what you offer, such as point-of-care documentation, order entry, automated medication dispensing, etc.
88. Take a highly personal approach to interviewing and talking with candidates at the recruiter and manager level—involve senior nursing leaders.
89. Expand human resources recruitment services hours to evenings and weekends.
90. Partner the prospective recruit with a staff RN on the unit for a half-day.
91. Develop a sourcing calendar by month to ensure a continuous applicant flow.

92. Evaluate life cycle needs of applicants and offer the schedule and position that meets those needs.

93. Have the chief nurse executive send flowers to new RN hires, with a welcoming letter.

94. Send recruiters to healthcare facilities in the area that are laying off RNs.

95. Capitalize on staff dissatisfaction in competitor hospitals and use refer-a-friend bonuses to hire a number of RNs, once one or more has joined your staff.

96. Hold a welcome party on the unit for new hires, before the employee begins—the word will travel.

97. Provide a career coach for RNs who need a change—recruit internally.

98. Recruit in administrative areas—many staff members have relatives in healthcare and do not know about internal job openings.

99. Hold a raffle for staff who have referred a friend or give a large cash prize or trip to the employee who recruits the most new staff members.

100. Watch the competition and then do not do what they do— do it better. Be unique in your market.

PART III

Staying Power: Retention Strategies

CHAPTER 6

The Right Work Environment

INTRODUCTION

Maintaining the right working environment is essential for retaining nurses. What constitutes a positive work environment, and how can nursing administration and management ensure that it is positive?

Nurses consider multiple aspects of their work environment:

- Overall culture of the organization—What is it like to work in the environment? What is valued by the organization?
- Climate or ambience of their particular unit or department— The manager can greatly affect that climate.
- Stress levels, and strategies for reducing stress.
- Staffing ratios, flexibility, and schedule adjustments that will allow them to be successful in both their professional and private lives.

Each of these areas is addressed below and are the focus of this chapter.

ORGANIZATIONAL CULTURE

Leininger (1991) defines organizational culture as the aims, norms, values, and practices of an organization in which people have goals and try to achieve them in beneficial ways. In other words, organizational culture is the organization's preferred ways of accomplishing goals, determining priorities, and making decisions. It affects not only people working in the institution, such as employees and volunteers, but also customers, such as physicians and patients.

Four types of organizational culture have been described in the literature. The *human resource perspective* describes a culture that strives to facilitate the fit between person and organization. When conflict arises, the solution considers the needs of the individual or group as well as the needs of the organization. The *political perspective* describes a culture that emphasizes power and politics. Problems are viewed as "turf" issues and are resolved by developing networks to increase the power base. In the *structural perspective* culture, the organization focuses on following rules or protocols. This culture relies on its policies and procedures to resolve conflict. The *symbolic perspective* culture relies on rituals, ceremony, and myths in determining appropriate behaviors. More than one culture may exist in an organization. For example, both human resource and symbolic perspectives may guide an organization.

Schein (1985) has used a tree analogy of leaves, trunk, and roots to describe organizational culture. Leaves represent the artifacts of the institution. This is what is seen and heard in the institution. For example, signage, pictures, interior design, dress code, traffic flow, medical equipment, and visible interactions are all visual leaves. Audible leaves would include languages spoken, stories, myths, and other conversations. The trunk represents the values: what is good, what is right, and what is true. The roots represent the assumptions. Assumptions define the culture of the organization. Because assumptions are invisible, they may not be recognized. At times, assumptions are ambiguous and self-contradictory. This may be the case especially when a merger or acquisition has occurred.

When attempting to recruit and retain nurses, it is critical for administration to consider how the organizational culture affects nurses. While an organization's culture is not inherently good or bad, or right or wrong, it may in subtle ways lend to decreases in the pool of nurses who select that organization. Therefore, healthcare institution recruiters should consider the fit between the organization and potential employees, and leaders should strive to promote a culture that reflects the human resource perspective. Nurses and other staff members in general need a culturally caring organization. Such organizations provide stability and incorporate universal care constructs, including respect for and about, concern for, and help and assistance to its employees. A thorough assessment of organizational culture is a helpful tool for senior management. It can be conducted using the Leininger Culture Care Universality and Diversity Model, as summarized in Figure 6.1.

CLIMATE

The nurse manager plays an important role in fostering a positive environment and developing and maintaining a cohesive social group that includes affiliation, friendship, a sense of group, and peer acknowledgment. Although difficult to quantify, such an environment is known to increase nursing staff satisfaction. Specific aspects of a positive climate described below include fostering fun, celebrating successes and looking for the bright side, respecting staff, and maintaining contact with all shifts.

Fostering Fun

Good work relationships can be fostered through fun, food, and humor. Nursing administrators who promote a fun atmosphere will be positively viewed by staff. Potluck lunches are always well-received and work especially well with culturally diverse staffs. For

Figure 6.1: Questions to Guide a Thorough Organizational Climate Assessment

Factor	Types of Questions
Environmental context	What is the general environment of the community that surrounds the organization? Socioeconomic status? Race/ethnicity? Emphasis on health? Living arrangements? Access to social services? Employment? Proximity to other health facilities?
Language and ethnohistory	What languages are spoken within the institution? By employees? By patients? How formal or informal are the lines of communication? How hierarchical? What communication strategies are used within the institution: Written? Posters? Electronic? Oral? Grapevine? How did the institution come to be? What was the original mission? How has it changed over the years?
Technology	How is technology used in the institution? Who uses it? Is patient documentation electronic? Is electronic order entry in place? Is the technology in place in the emergency department, critical care units, labor and delivery, radiology, surgical suites, etc. cutting edge? Is e-mail used? Is web-based technology embraced?
Religious/ philosophical	Does the institution have a religious affiliation? Are religious symbols displayed within the facility? By patients? By staff? Is the institution private or public? For-profit or not-for-profit?
Kinship and social factors	What are the working relationships within nursing? Between nursing and ancillary services? Between nursing and medicine? How closely are staff members aligned?

Figure 6.1: *(continued)*

Factor	Types of Questions
Kinship and social factors *(continued)*	Is the environment emotionally warm and close or cold and distant? How do employees relate to each other? Do they celebrate together? Turn to each other for support? Do employees get together outside of work?
Cultural values	Are values explicitly stated? What is valued within the institution? What is viewed as good? What is viewed as right? What is seen as truth?
Political/legal	How politically charged is the institution? Where does the power rest within the institution? With medicine? With finance? With nursing? Is power shared? What types of legal actions have been taken against the institution? On behalf of the institution?
Economic	What is the financial viability of the institution? Who makes the financial decisions? How do the salaries and benefits compare to competitors in the immediate environment?
Educational	How is education valued within the institution? What type of assistance (financial, scheduling, flexibility) is provided for staff seeking advanced degrees? Does the institution provide education for medicine, nursing, and other professions? Are advanced practice nurses utilized? What is the educational background of staff nurses? Nurse managers? Nursing leaders? How does this compare to education of other professional groups? To competing organizations?

Source: Leininger (1996).

example, managers can ask nurses to bring foods that represent their cultural group to share with the department. This helps nurses recognize and appreciate other cultural groups and builds team thinking. To keep snacks healthy, managers may provide fresh fruit or air-popped popcorn periodically. This will provide a welcome relief to typical high-fat and high-sugar coffee-break foods and will help show the nurses how much they are appreciated. Fun activities outside of work, such as bowling, softball, and meals, can also be planned at the department level.

Observing special occasions on the unit adds fun to the day, fosters a positive work environment, and recognizes nurses as people. Be sure the managers are inclusive. Do not celebrate one person's birthday and not another's. Instead, managers can suggest a monthly birthday celebration and keep celebrations short, so nurses are not inconvenienced. Celebrate special birthdays like a critical care RN's 70th birthday with much fanfare; invite physicians, administration, and other staff associates. For other recognition efforts, prepare a basket of small gifts, such as calming teas and lotions, tapes, and gift certificates for videos, coffee, and bookstore purchases. Having the chief nurse executive (CNE) bring the basket is particularly effective as a recognition strategy. Provide many ideas for managers to use that will recognize staff and make work fun.

Senior nursing leaders and the CNE can liven up Nurses' Week by holding raffles for "home-grown" prizes. The CNE could offer a catered lunch in the administrative area for ten RNs or could prepare breakfast on the unit. An RN could win "CNE for a Day" privileges, a director could function as a nursing assistant, or a catered picnic could be another raffle prize.

An easy way to have fun on the unit and help nurses get to know one another is to suggest a "secret pal" exchange. Each nurse writes on a slip of paper his or her name, birthday, and a short list of things he or she enjoys. For example, one RN may list chocolate, reading, travel, and dogs, whereas another may list cooking, theater, and mountain climbing. The slips of paper are placed in a container.

Each person picks one, making sure no one selects himself or herself. Each nurse then becomes the secret pal of the nurse whose name he or she has drawn. During a short period of time (perhaps two weeks or a month), the nurse's mission is to do something creative, spontaneous, and fun for the secret pal. For example, a secret pal could give the nurse who likes chocolate, reading, travel, and dogs a piece of chocolate, travel information from the Internet about an exotic location, or a paperback book about dogs. The intent is not to spend money but to help staff get to know each other and do something special for him or her. Identities need to be kept secret. Allow staff to have fun with this, and at the end of the specified time, have a get-together where secret pals are revealed. Staff will enjoy coming up with creative ways to surprise their colleagues and will enjoy getting to know a little more about each other. This is an effective strategy your managers can use to make the workplace fun.

Another way for staff to get to know each other and lift morale is to ask nurses to bring in pictures of themselves as babies for posting on a bulletin board. Everyone will enjoy looking at the pictures and trying to match photo with nurse. Even patients, families, and physicians can join in.

The manager can also build unit spirit by using symbols. For example, the manager can ask staff nurses to come up with a unit or group slogan and logo. Nurses can be encouraged to design a lapel pin, a t-shirt, or a unit poster. This positive group identity will help build enthusiasm. It will also highlight the distinctiveness of your staff and unit.

Gentle humor can help build enthusiasm as well. For example, the manager might keep a "Tickle Me Elmo" toy in the workstation. When a nurse is having a particularly hard day, she gets the toy. When Elmo laughs hysterically while being tickled, most people cannot help but join in the laughter.

To help retain nurses, managers need to encourage staff to take time off. Be sure to take time off yourself to set an example for your managers. Nurses who feel they can never take vacations are likely to burn out much more quickly than those who do. In addition, nurses who are overworked, stressed, and tired are a liability to the unit. Nurses need downtime and preventive maintenance or they will burn out. Watch out for managers and RNs with excessive vacation time owed them—chances are they need to take it.

Celebrating Successes and Looking for the Bright Side

The nurse manager must always celebrate successes. This helps team members find joy in work even in this era of high census, high acuity, and scarce resources. Successes are any events, changes, or behaviors that show your organization is moving toward its vision and acting in concert with its values. The changes may be incremental (e.g., all physicians located their charts today) or more significant (e.g., all patients with DRG 089 received their antibiotic within four hours this week). Posting letters from satisfied customers (patients, families, physicians, and others) is another way to celebrate successes. In addition, the manager should broadcast and publish nurse and unit successes as part of the positive environment. Details should be given to both administration and public relations.

Even when things go wrong, the manager can set the pace by looking for the bright side and use it to coach staff. It is important to help nurses see opportunities rather than stumble over obstacles and challenges. It is possible to draw something good from every situation. For example, a patient fall can result in changes in unit procedures and increased patient safety. The effective manager helps nurses see this big picture and the contributions they are making to it.

Respecting Staff

Nurse managers should look for the "unofficial" leaders of the nursing unit. These informal leaders have a tremendous impact on the unit's day-to-day functioning and relationships. Enlist these nurses to welcome new members to the staff and integrate new members into the work group. Excluding new staff members is a sure way to affect retention long term. Instead, move forward as a cohesive group. Remember that talented people will not tolerate disrespect for long. To keep good people, it is critical that they are shown respect in consistent ways and recognized for their unique qualities.

Celebrating individual differences is another crucial way of showing respect. Diversity of talent and perspectives strengthens a work group. However, differences may also get in the way. How do you ensure that managers are celebrating, not just tolerating, differences? A first step is to ask managers to look at their own beliefs. How much do they respect nurses who are different from them? Do they value what the differences bring to their team?

To help truly celebrate diversity, begin by analyzing your own attitudes and prejudices. Admit to your leanings toward or away from those with different skin color, status, education, height, weight, title, accent, sexual orientation, or geographic origin. Then notice how your prejudices play out at work. Whom did you last promote? Whom do you tend to ignore, praise less often, or be friendly toward? Third, make a conscious decision to change. Practice fairness, and consciously avoid discriminating. These steps will help you appreciate and use individual strengths, styles, and talents. You will also serve as a role model for staff.

Maintaining Contact with All Shifts

Always be sure to keep in touch with off-shift nurses and encourage nursing leadership to do the same. This will foster communication across the shifts and assure staff that you know how important nurses are around the clock. Encourage your managers to come in early one day a week to interact with those on nights and to stay late periodically to talk with those on the afternoon and evening shifts. Make rounds; leave your office door open. Ask managers to plan staff meetings so that nurses from all shifts are able to attend. This might mean having several department meetings, or videotaping the meetings and making the videotape and minutes available for review. Be sure to keep track of attendance to the meetings. When certain staff nurses are not attending, the managers should invite them and include them by letting them know that their input is valuable. If they continue to resist involvement, let them know management's expectations regarding attendance.

Also, be sure to involve nurses from all shifts in task forces and committees. This broadens understanding and involvement. Consistently send the message that the nurses are integral to the unit and nursing department and can improve it. Demonstrate that you trust them and respect their ideas and judgment. Show them how their good ideas can be implemented.

Plan to visit staff and bring goodies for at least one holiday a year. Senior nursing leaders or managers with a cart of holiday cookies and punch taken unit to unit is good for morale and provides visibility on off shifts. This helps nurses to understand you are thinking of them. Some nurse managers and directors work holidays occasionally to keep in touch and see how the department functions. Be sure to attend shift parties or functions when asked. This is a great opportunity to get to know nurses better and to learn about the challenges they face on their shift.

STRESS LEVELS

Nursing leadership should be aware of the stresses inherent in nursing practice and should be able to determine how to support the staff in difficult situations and how to be sure that staff know the variety of support mechanisms available. Staff should be encouraged to take advantage of employee health and wellness programs offered by the healthcare organization.

Reducing Stress Levels Overall

The nurse manager can help to reduce work stress in a number of ways. First, nurses need to know what is expected of them in their jobs. In addition, nurses need sufficient orientation and adequate training. Specific detail must be provided on performance standards, company policies, codes of personal conduct, required procedures, and expected performance outcomes. Nurses need to be allowed and encouraged to raise concerns and problems about their work, and a process must be in place to address and resolve these concerns. Unacceptable behaviors must be fairly and consistently addressed. Poor work must not be tolerated, and good work must be recognized and rewarded.

In addition, nurses must be aware of their personal performances—both areas of strength and areas for improvement. Nurses need to be helped to develop internal assessments of their own performance, and not just rely on your external evaluation. Supportive, coaching relationships must be fostered. For example, new nurses should be paired with experienced nurses who are good at mentoring new RNs.

Nurses need some control over their work processes. When possible, allow nurses to determine how and when to perform an action. Create a climate of improvement by encouraging all nurses to share their ideas and suggestions. Show them you value their thoughts and opinions. Encourage the formation of ad hoc teams to address nursing unit, overall nursing, and organizational problems. Be sure to follow up with every team that submits a suggestion and see what can be done to implement it. Reward the suggestions that result in improvement. Praise the group in front of peers or take the nurse team out to lunch to recognize a job well done.

Nurse managers should also be encouraged to foster wellness. Lectures, employee assistance programs, flu shots, fitness classes or access to fitness centers, smoking cessation programs, weight loss programs, cardiac risk assessment evaluations, and counseling centers are a few programs that may be offered by employers to help employees stay well. Self-care is also important. Nurses need time off for renewal to do things that are important to them. Ensuring adequate time off that is protected from constant telephone calls to return to work sends a powerful message to staff that their wellness is important.

Identifying and Modifying Major Contributors to Stress

Several issues can affect stress levels, thus having a major impact on retention. These issues include poor team relationships, strained physician-nurse relations, and problematic staff members. These must be recognized and addressed. Each issue is discussed below.

Poor Team Relationships

A dysfunctional work team, strained colleague relations, or poor management-to-staff relations can lead to turnover and job dissatisfaction. You may have a warning that team relationships are dysfunctional if you see several of the indicators below:

- Complaints to the human resources department
- High turnover
- Poor employee satisfaction survey results
- Few internal transfers because of negative perceptions
- Negative exit interview data

Signs and symptoms should be taken seriously and an action plan developed that is based on the source of the dissatisfaction. If you see increased turnover, but the cause is unknown, the situation should be investigated. Several strategies follow:

- Have human resources or a facilitator external to the unit conduct focus groups of staff and one-on-one interviews with unit leadership personnel.
- Use brainstorming, structured discussion, and open-ended questions to ensure input.
- Try posting questions or using electronic mail to invite staff working evenings, nights, and weekends to provide input on a 24-hour-a-day and 7-day-a-week basis.
- Develop and implement a plan based on issues identified by the staff. Be sure that a way to monitor progress, such as turnover rate, is built into the plan.

Strained Physician-Nurse Relations

If physician-nurse relations are at the heart of a dissatisfied nursing staff, take quick action. Gain sponsorship from medical and nursing leadership to address issues organizationally, departmentally, or at the unit level. A skilled facilitator may be needed, depending on the situation. Begin by focusing on one area, such as improving communication, addressing patient care issues, enhancing collaboration, or addressing specific process issues. Medical leadership and willing participants are necessary for the initiative to be successful. A communication plan for nurses and physicians should also be developed.

Problematic Staff Member(s)

The observant manager will be aware of problematic staff members and should address them proactively. The manager must observe, listen to staff feedback, and identify themes in customer complaints. One-to-one counseling with specific behavioral and job performance expectations should be put in writing for the staff. Poor staff morale often results when poor performance and negative behavior and attitudes are allowed to continue. The manager must educate or replace, or prepare to fail. Keeping negative staff with problematic behaviors is a recipe for disaster.

Each of these situations exhausts and demoralizes nursing staff. Team relationship issues must be addressed. If they are not resolved, retention efforts will not likely be successful—staff will speak with their feet.

Addressing Nursing Burnout

Nurse burnout, which is prevalent in the hospital workplace, has a major impact on retention and should be identified and addressed. Nurses often minimize the stress inherent in their daily lives, and such inattention may result in nurses leaving their current job or leaving the profession altogether. Colleagues, family members, or friends are often the first to notice the change in behavior. Warning signs of nursing burnout include:

- forgetfulness
- appetite increase or decrease
- insomnia
- depression or anxiety
- dysfunctional relationships
- frequent illnesses or episodes of calling in sick
- cynical or withdrawn behavior
- stress or tension headaches

Nurses may feel emotionally drained or exhausted and may "depersonalize" care, which manifests itself in an uncaring or callous attitude. They may feel a lack of personal accomplishment or feel worthless. Strategies for addressing nurse burnout are presented in the next section.

Strategies for Preventing Burnout and Reducing Stress

Interdisciplinary Patient Care Conferences

Interdisciplinary patient care conferences allow nurses to interact with social workers, pastoral caregivers, physicians, family members, and other nurses to address and clarify difficult issues. These conferences continue the dialog and invite input from the RN, which increases the nurse's role in decision making and enhances his or her sense of importance to the patient care team.

Peer Support/Forums

Informal discussion among colleagues is very important. The support, guidance, and sensitivity provided by a colleague is in itself a powerful antidote for stress. Grief support groups, case review, and discussion groups with a trained facilitator should be used.

Ethics Consultations

Nurses should be able to access an ethics consultant or hospital ethics committee to assist in ethical dilemmas that have few, if any, answers. Ethics education is also important.

Still Points

A "still point" is a time during the day when RNs can go to a quiet place for meditation and spiritual renewal. The setting should be relaxing; it may be a chapel, a garden, or a similar place of beauty and tranquility. The environment should be calm, quiet, and away from the unit.

Critical Incident Stress Management Debriefings

During a critical incident stress management debriefing, specially trained staff are deployed to assist other staff or the community in dealing with difficult situations, such as a mass casualty event, a pediatric trauma, or child abuse. Nurses should be free to access these services as needed based on their clinical practice.

Employee Assistance Programs

Confidential employee assistance programs are helpful as nurses deal with both job and personal stress. Mandatory referrals or self-referrals can provide RNs with much-needed support in coping with stress in their work or personal lives. Difficult personal situations spill over into work life, and coping mechanisms are needed that will affect both.

Care for the Caregiver Sessions

Organizational, departmental, or clinical unit "care for the caregiver" sessions can be tailored to specific needs. Stress reduction techniques can be taught; stress reduction kits with candles, lotions, aromatherapy, herbal teas, and other soothing items can be provided for staff; and 15-minute back and neck massages can be offered in a break room.

A care plan for stress is outlined in Figure 6.2. Deep breathing is one effective technique that is easily used in almost any setting.

FLEXIBLE SCHEDULING AND LIFESTYLE OPTIONS

Specific strategies to retain RNs should be focused on flexible staffing and scheduling, adequate staffing, and autonomy. In addition, strategies ensuring that nurses have a "voice" in their nursing practice

Figure 6.2: Peak Performance Enhancement Through Breathing, Relaxation, and Meditation—A Care Plan for Stress

Stress comes from many sources. Sometimes stress happens when we are excited or looking forward to something. Other times we worry about losing things that are important to us. There are occasions when a traumatic incident has caused an abrupt change. At times we feel like it is difficult to trust the routines and rhythms of our lives. Each of these circumstances can cause a predictable emotional response that we call *stress*. Identifying how you feel can help you to understand what has caused your experience of stress.

You know when you are performing well. You might say you're "in the zone" or "in the groove." Similarly, you know when you're not performing as well. You might say you're "out of synch" or "out of rhythm."

When you perform at the peak of your ability, your mind and body work in harmony with very little visible effort. At this level of performance, the mind and body work as one. You are not thinking about the things that the brain needs to do because they are happening naturally and automatically.

When you experience anxiety, the mind begins to problem solve which, unfortunately, reduces access to memory. At times, the anxiety creates its own panic and prediction of failure, which generates additional stress. This stress response can happen before or during a challenging task or activity. When the stress response occurs, over 1,400 physiological changes are activated that result in subtracting from your performance. When one of these physical changes occurs, the others follow.

Learning to calm your body and clear your thoughts before and during a challenging task or activity helps you bring your mind and body into harmony. This can be accomplished through a simple series of breathing, relaxation, and meditation exercises.

Breathing: *Take a series of three deep breaths, first emptying your lungs of air, then inhaling slowly through your nose, allowing the air to fill your stomach. Breathe out slowly through your mouth, allowing the exhale to last twice as long as the inhale (e.g. inhale for two seconds; exhale for four, then 3/6, then 4/8). Make sure that you are breathing with your diaphragm (stomach goes out when you inhale) rather than your chest.*

(continued)

Figure 6.2 *(continued)*

Relaxation: *Beginning at the top of your head, locate each muscle group in your body, moving slowly from head to neck to torso to extremities. As you find each muscle, tense it for a period of two seconds as you inhale diaphragmatically, then allow it to completely relax for four seconds as you slowly exhale. Imagine the tension leaving your body as you gradually move through each muscle group with each breath until you have tensed and relaxed each muscle from head to toe.*

Meditation: *Choose a pleasant word or visual image that you can hear and see in your imagination. Think of this word or image every time you exhale for about 15 minutes each day. If you have an intrusive thought or feeling during your meditation, return to the repetition of your relaxing word or image. Use this word or image during your task or activity to return your mind and body to harmony.*

Source: Reprinted with permission from the Advocate Lutheran General Hospital Mental Health Division, 2000, Park Ridge, Illinois.

are important. They must have enablers to allow more time in patient care and less time on administrative and clerical issues. Providing mentors and preceptors and rewarding those in these roles, along with effective leadership and supervision, are equally as important as a competitive wage and benefit program.

Flexible Scheduling

Adequate staffing and flexible scheduling are among the top retention strategies in most surveys conducted within the industry. Flexible staffing schedules help provide staff with the work-life balance sought throughout the career continuum. Offering control over hours and shifts worked, with many flexible options, consistently proves critical in today's competitive environment. Conducting focus groups to identify your staff's needs is a necessary step in developing flexible options. Organizations that offer a variety of flexible work options, such as permanent shifts, part-time shifts, night incentive programs, weekend programs, 12-hour shifts, and flex-time, to meet lifestyle needs will consistently retain RNs.

The following scheduling options may be considered:

36 for 40. RNs work three 12-hour shifts (36 hours) and are paid for 40 hours and receive full-time benefits. An alternative is to pay for 36 hours and offer full-time benefits.

Weekend program. Weekend-only staff options meet a number of needs, including requiring fewer weekends of regular staff and providing weekend shifts for staff who have child care or other responsibilities that create the demand for a weekend-only schedule. Staff may work Friday and Saturday or Saturday and Sunday on 12-hour shifts, or Friday, Saturday, and Sunday on 8-hour shifts. A weekend differential of $5 to $10 per hour is paid, on top of any existing weekend rotating premium. A minimum of a six-month commitment that is renewable is required, with the option of returning to vacant staff positions. Compensation is built in as an hourly premium or into base salary.

Night life program. Night life programs offer permanent shifts and additional compensation for those who can make a minimum of a six-month to one-year commitment. This decreases or eliminates the need for regular staff rotation to nights, which markedly enhances staff satisfaction. An additional shift incentive may be added for each shift, or the RN may receive the compensation at the end of the renewable commitment period.

Resource RN. RNs with two or more years of experience may be assigned throughout a division, such as adult critical care, medical/surgical, or women's and children's services, or in smaller facilities housewide to enhance staffing. Family medical leaves, illness, paid time off, and vacancies significantly affect staffing. Resource RNs, with their flexibility and willingness to work in several units, are an invaluable asset to an organization. The resource RN may receive a variety of incentives, including permanent shifts, up to a 20 percent higher rate of pay, fewer weekends, and self-scheduling. These employees may be full- or part-time and receive benefits.

PRN or per diem. Non-benefits-eligible RNs who receive a premium pay rate are an important staffing resource, and the flexibility this offers may meet a lifestyle need for some nurses. These staff members either provide their availability or are offered available shifts after schedules are completed. A commitment to a minimum amount of duty should be required, usually one shift per week, with additional requirements for holidays, off shifts, and weekend shifts. Salaries are generally higher for these positions because no benefits are offered.

Winter hours. A 9-month option, with three months off during the summer, for example, may be desirable if it meets the needs of patient care. This schedule works best in seasonal environments where the overall population increases in the winter months, or in the pediatric mental health arena if the census is higher in the winter months. A 12-month contract as an exempt employee, or a 9-month salary divided over 12 months, are compensation options.

Organizations that offer great flexibility in their scheduling options over the career continuum for the RN will retain most effectively. New graduates have different needs than the mid- or late-career RN; parents of small children have different needs than do those caring for ill or elderly relatives.

Lifestyle Options

Other benefits that are important to work-life balance are flexible benefits, with tuition reimbursement ranking in the top half in most retention surveys. In addition, continuing education, healthcare insurance, retirement savings plans, and paid time off are frequently cited as important benefit features that keep RNs on the job.

Working in a partnership with nurses to provide flexible schedules will enhance your desirability as an employer of choice. Enablers are also important to staff so they can meet scheduling and staffing needs. The following are some examples of enablers:

- on-site or near-site child care that is open early and with evening hours, based on needs assessment
- days off for school, special occasions, and other personal needs, granted in advance
- a resource and referral center for child care and older adult care
- emergency loans and assistance in times of crisis
- paid time off donation to a central bank or to those who have depleted their hours because of a family or health crisis

STAFFING/WORKLOAD OPTIONS THAT CONTRIBUTE TO RETENTION

Adequate staffing is one of the retention factors mentioned most often by RNs. Nurse-to-patient ratios are a political issue from coast to coast; mandated staffing ratios are required in California and pending in several other states. Nurses want to be able to spend time with their patients and offer the compassion and competent skilled nursing care that drew them to the nursing profession.

Nurse-to-patient ratios have eroded during the past few years as a result of managed care, declining reimbursement, reengineering, and cost management. Assuring RNs of adequate staffing ratios is important in recruitment and retention. Adequate ratios vary by type of facility, shift, acuity, and availability.

RNs have been viewed as a variable resource, and past practice has been to call off RNs or send them home early when census drops. This practice affects retention negatively and is not recommended. Instead, staff should be used in a variety of other ways:

- They may be cross-trained and floated to other units in which they are competent.
- They may complete self-directed continuing education.
- They may develop education modules.

- They may collect data for infection control, quality assurance, and quality improvement activities.

These roles are limited only by our ability to conceptualize them.

Reducing a nurse's income in an unpredictable way over time is a sure way to motivate staff to seek employment elsewhere. Instead, consider guaranteeing a 40-hour work week, like the program being piloted at Kaiser Permanente's three South Bay Hospitals. Rather than canceling shifts when patient volume is low, nurses at the three hospitals (San Jose, Santa Clara, and Redwood City) are given other duties, such as filling in for nurses on break, doing administration work, or getting additional training. The hospitals estimate the cost to recruit one nurse to be $40,000. The Kaiser hour-guarantee program costs $1.6 million. If the hospital retains 40 nurses as a result of this policy change, the cost of the program will be offset. Programs like this demonstrate respect for nurses.

Staffing Patterns

Staffing appropriately may be approached simplistically, based on staffing grids in which the number of RNs and other caregivers needed and available are developed by nursing leadership, with exceptions specified to the degree possible. For example, assume a 1:5 RN-to-patient ratio is recommended for the medical/surgical unit. If one patient has a cardiac arrest while more than 15 telemetry patients are on the unit and more than 5 are post-ICU patients, these factors may change the ratio to 1:4. When ratios are developed in collaboration with the nursing leadership team and staff at the unit level, the buy-in is much better than when using an arbitrary finance target. Patient acuity systems also may be used to allocate staff appropriately by service. (Patient acuity systems are used to identify the patient's severity of illness for the purpose of predicting nursing care hours required.) A pitfall in many acuity-based systems is the inability to actually staff to the levels recommended, thus creating distrust in the acuity system. Again, using staff RNs and the leadership team in the development of the standards is a critical success factor in the acceptance of the system. A number of commercial systems are available, or the acuity system can be developed internally.

National benchmarks of nursing hours per patient day may be obtained from state hospital associations, from legislative ratios in mandated RN-to-patient ratio states, and from publications ranking the top 100 hospitals, consulting firms, management engineering society databases, and other sources. Benchmarking with similar hospitals will provide data on appropriate nurse-to-patient ratios. Ratios vary by shift, clinical unit, size of hospital, type of hospital, and availability of RNs, LPNs or LVNs, and RN extenders. The easiest way to compare ratios is with your colleagues at similar hospitals or by using local or state databases within hospital associations.

The California-mandated ratios passed in 1999 are expected to be enacted in 2003. Proposed ratios from the office of California governor Gray Davis are shown in Figure 6.3.

Understaffing

Understaffing is common in many hospitals because of vacancies in budgeted positions, sick calls, vacations, family medical leaves, orientation, and continuing education. Hospitals should have written guidelines that govern how they provide safe patient care. A variety of methods may be used to cover understaffing. These methods include the following:

- using an admission RN to do all admissions for the shift
- using an in-house float pool or "occasional" staff to cover problematic shifts
- using RNs to float from another unit in which competencies enable them to provide care to patients
- requesting overtime from full-time staff or additional hours from part-time staff

Figure 6.3: California's Proposed Minimum Nurse-Staffing Ratios

Hospital Unit	Proposed Nurse-to-Patient Ratio
Intensive/critical care unit	1:2
Operating room	1:1
Neonatal ICU	1:2
Intermediate-care nursery	1:4
Well-baby nursery	1:8
Postpartum	1:8 (1:4 couplets)
(when multiple births, the number of	1:6 (mothers only)
newborns and mothers shall not exceed	
eight per nurse)	
Labor and delivery	1:2
Post-anesthesia care unit	1:2
Emergency department	1:4
Critical care	1:2
Trauma	1:1
Burn unit	1:2
Pediatrics	1:4
Step-down/telemetry	1:4
Specialty care (oncology)	1:5
Telemetry unit	1:5
General medical/surgical	1:6 (initial)
	1:5 (to be phased in)
Behavioral health psychiatric units	1:6
Mixed units	1:6 (initial)
	1:5 (to be phased in)

Note: At the time of publication, the California Nurses Association reports, "the ratios must still be finalized following a public comment period." Please visit www.calnurse.org for updates.

Source: California AB 394, 1999; California Nurses Association (2001).

- asking RNs to move from better-staffed shifts to the problematic shifts
- using "call in" or "on call" staff; this is part of the RN employment agreement

- using personnel from the leadership team who have appropriate competencies to work additional shifts
- using external RN agencies that demonstrate competencies to meet patient care needs and are able to provide documented evidence of meeting regulatory requirements
- using a resource RN, whose job it is to float to a variety of units

Mandatory overtime should be used only as a last resort. This is well-documented as a major nurse dissatisfier and will lead to RN turnover if used consistently as a staffing tool.

Staffing Incentives

A variety of staffing incentives can be used for hard-to-fill shifts or areas. These incentives will help you avoid mandatory overtime and provide safe patient care. Optimally, if recruitment and retention strategies are used that work, incentives will be unnecessary. Some incentives include the following:

- Staff sign up for designated on-call shifts and receive on-call pay; if needed, they are called in to work a particular shift.
- PRN or occasional staff, who receive a premium rate of pay without benefits, are used to fill in on hard-to-fill shifts after regular staff receive their assignments.
- Bonus payments are given to RNs who work when not scheduled, ranging from $25 per shift to double pay.
- Part-time staff agree to work extra hours for a designated period of time and receive an incentive bonus payment at the end of the period.
- Staff agree to work additional hard-to-fill hours for double-time pay.

- Cross-trained RNs serve as resource nurses and receive a premium rate of pay and full-time benefits in exchange for being available to staff wherever they are needed.

Alternative Strategies for Short Staffing

In addition to staff incentives, other strategies to solve staffing shortages include reducing the number of staffed beds, declining transfers or transports from other hospitals, delaying or canceling elective admissions and procedures, and diverting emergency cases to other hospitals by following state protocols. All of these strategies should be used as a last resort, because they affect referral patterns and customer satisfaction and may negatively affect hospital revenues.

SUMMARY

This chapter has covered a variety of topics related to the work environment necessary for retaining nurses. Organizational culture is central to how the institution is perceived by nurses and affects both the retention and recruitment of nursing staff. Fostering a positive climate is an essential obligation for managers and others within an institution. Nurses will resign if they are not respected and if positive relationships are not fostered. Managers must monitor stress levels and mitigate them as needed. Strategies for reducing stress and burnout must be in place to provide a positive working environment. Flexible scheduling and lifestyle options must be provided to staff, and these options may need to change over time as nursing staff members' needs change. Last, staffing and workload must be considered.

The right work environment is a necessary component of nursing staff retention. The next chapter will describe why career growth and professional development are other essential components for retention.

REFERENCES

California Nurses Association. 2001. "AB 394: California and the Demand for Safe and Effective Nurse to Patient Ratios." Report. [Online report; retrieved Feb. 2002.] www.calnurse.org/cna/nrsptrt/ihspab394.pdf.

Leininger, M. 1996. "Founder's Focus. Transcultural Nursing Administration: An Imperative Worldwide." *Journal of Transcultural Nursing* 8 (1): 28–33.

———. 1991. *Culture Care Diversity and Universality: A Theory of Nursing Care.* New York: National League for Nursing Press.

Schein, E.H. 1985. *Organizational Culture and Leadership.* San Francisco: Jossey-Bass.

CHAPTER 7

Career Growth and Professional Development

INTRODUCTION

Career advancement and development are very important to nurses. Many RNs do not wish to move into management but want other advancement opportunities. Advancement opportunities in education, management, advanced clinical specialization, and nontraditional positions that require a nursing background are of interest, along with advancement at the bedside.

Healthcare environments should address this fundamental need by considering what the RN needs and wants that is compatible with what the organization needs, wants, and can afford. Career advancement options are numerous and are based on resource availability, funding, and staff interest.

The organization that creates an environment in which professional development is continuous throughout the RN's career, beginning with orientation, will retain its staff. Mentoring and precepting can improve recognition and retention. "Grow your own" programs will ensure a continuous supply of new graduates and specialty RNs. Promotion of nursing through word and deed demonstrates to nurses and to the organization the value of nursing.

LIFELONG LEARNING

Lifelong learning is a very powerful motivator for RNs, and the organization that fosters continuous learning will retain its staff. Promoting self-assessment by recognizing and reinforcing what the nurse is doing, providing a road map for the RN for professional development, and enabling the RN to enhance his or her critical thinking skills are simple, inexpensive ways to build loyalty with your staff.

Fostering Self-assessment Skills

Encouraging nurses to recognize their own good performances is important. Nurses who acknowledge what they do well are more optimistic and confident when they face new challenges. Self-esteem is an important factor in this effort. A variety of techniques can be used to build self-esteem in staff. First, it is critical to give staff members only assignments they are capable of doing. As they become more proficient, their responsibilities should be increased. In addition, the manager should only offer help in the form of added training and support if the nurse needs it. Otherwise, allow the nurse to figure out the solution or correct process. Do not micromanage, or make decisions that are best handled by a subordinate, as this technique only reinforces the image of incompetence. When you as the boss are involved in making all of the decisions, second guessing the nurses' judgment, or establishing a permission-seeking environment for even the smallest issues, the RN will not achieve the confidence he or she needs to feel successful.

Managers should give positive reinforcement for achievements. Recognize nurses for what they have done, recognize their suggestions, complement them on their meeting contributions, ask them for advice, praise progress, and thank them for their help.

Managers must help nurses identify their own strengths and accomplishments. One easy way to do this is to have managers distribute blank sheets of paper at a meeting or training session. The nurses should be asked to list the five most exceptional things they have done at work in the past year. Encourage them to list anything they did that was above expectations or might seem remarkable to others if they knew about it. Staff keep their own lists and may volunteer to read them. While this exercise can be presented as a fun warm-up for meetings, it has a serious side as well. It generates fun and laughter while it builds self-confidence and optimism, which are linked with the ability to motivate oneself.

As an alternative, each nurse can create a success folder. Everyone receives a brightly colored folder marked "My Successes." They jot down all the positive feedback they get verbally from you, coworkers, physicians, patients, and others on their work. These notes should be placed in the file. Nurses should also store positive e-mails, notes, and memos in the folder. When they become temporarily discouraged, the manager encourages them to pull out the file and look at their accomplishments.

Building an RN Road Map

Managers should always talk to staff about their careers, and are responsible for beginning the dialog. They should listen for information that will tell them more about the nurses. Questions need to be asked that will help staff think about their unique skills, interests, and values. The conversation is meaningful to staff, and the answers will provide information to help managers partner with staff as they manage their own careers. Questions such as the following can be used by the managers:

- What makes you unique to this organization?
- Tell me about an accomplishment of which you are particularly proud.
- Are your interests being met here? In what ways?

Figure 7.1: Example of an RN Road Map

Kendall is a new RN who has been heavily recruited by four local hospitals. Sign-on bonuses, night shift differentials, premium pay, and promises of low patient-to-RN ratios have been offered. Kendall is confused; the hospitals all seem alike to her. Kendall sees a reasonable salary and benefits package as a given. She expects to work undesirable hours in the beginning. All offers appear to be the same.

Kendall has one last interview at a hospital on the outskirts of the city. From the start, it is different from her other interviews. The recruiter asks Kendall what matters most to her as she starts her career. Kendall tells the recruiter her hopes and aspirations for her nursing career. The recruiter asks where she hopes to be in five years. Kendall indicates she would like to be an oncology advanced practice nurse or a nurse researcher in oncology. Kendall also tells the recruiter how important community outreach is to her. The recruiter suggests they map out a career path for Kendall that will allow her to reach her goal.

The path starts in a general medical unit for one year, with orientation, continuing education, and a mentor. A career coach, an oncology clinical nurse specialist, would be assigned to meet with Kendall monthly. Kendall would also attend several oncology educational offerings. In year two, Kendall

- What might enrich your current job?
- In what ways do you need to become more effective? How might you do that?
- What do you need to learn? How might you learn it?

Establishing a written career path or career road map is an ideal retention strategy for those nurses wishing to advance over time. The organization that provides this will have a unique positioning strategy in the market. Helping a nurse develop an individual road map may occur as early as recruitment (Figure 7.1).

Every nurse should have at least one development goal. It might be to take a course, learn a new skill, or give a presentation. Nurses would be transferred to the oncology unit when a position became available. She would be provided a thorough orientation to oncology. She would also enroll in graduate school part-time, using tuition assistance and flexible scheduling options. She would focus on oncology advanced practice nursing.

In years three and four, Kendall's career path would be validated. If oncology is still Kendall's desired path, additional education would be provided, including participation in a research project. Four continuing education days per year would be supported. In year five, when Kendall finished her degree, she could look at all available positions that met her needs. Should a position not be available, Kendall could take advantage of a career advancement program at the unit level.

Kendall debated very briefly. No sign-on bonus was offered, nor was a night bonus program offered; also very few openings were available. The drive from her home was 30 minutes each way. Yet Kendall really wanted the job. She had found the professional practice environment she was seeking. Kendall accepted the job and her career path evolved over time. Kendall became the bone marrow transplant advanced practice nurse, a career she loves. Many of her friends have yet to find the nursing career of their dreams.

who do not have a goal may need help coming up with one. Nurses who are always learning something new are more likely to be satisfied than those who feel they have stopped growing.

It is important to encourage staff to look at their overall balance. How much peace, fulfillment, contentment, and creativity are they experiencing in their life? A simple exercise is to have the manager ask each nurse to assess his or her energy level on a scale of 1 to 10. If the nurse scores below 5, chances are they are not experiencing fulfillment and their job is not energizing them. Knowing what motivates the nurse, what he or she wants to learn, and how he or she plans to practice in the future will help assist the nurse whose energy is depleted.

Stimulating Critical Thinking Skills

Managers should provide an environment that stimulates nurses' critical thinking skills. One way to do this is by having managers post on a flip chart or white board a realistic ethical situation that relates to the types of patients for which the nurses care. Two or three specific questions about the situation are included. Nurses are asked for their opinions about how to handle the posted situation by answering the questions. Answers should be viewed by other staff members, but not by patients. The scenario and responses can be discussed at your regular staff meeting. Someone from the ethics committee can attend to offer additional insight and discuss difficult ethical dilemmas with staff.

Another way to foster critical thinking is to have advanced practice nurses (APN) mentor staff at the bedside. APNs can also do nursing rounds or hold nursing grand rounds, similar to the format used by the medical staff.

PROVIDING EDUCATIONAL OPPORTUNITIES FOR NURSING STAFF

Ongoing education, an orientation program that focuses on results, self-directed learning, and a program in which RNs help educate other RN staff are important retention tools. Ongoing learning is important to most nurses, and sharing knowledge is a powerful staff motivation tool.

Orientation Programs

Experienced nurses sometimes have difficulty remembering being a new graduate or functioning in an unfamiliar environment. In addition to taking on the role of nurse in a new environment, new nurses must also develop collegial relationships with other nurses and learn the politics of the unit. Combined, these experiences are stressful by their very nature.

Orientation is the new hire's first experience with and impression of the organization. It sets the stage for how the RN feels about the organization and how well-prepared he or she is to begin practice. A new graduate has very different orientation needs than an experienced RN.

Cost-management initiatives often result in cuts in nursing education departments and ongoing education. This is the wrong place to make reductions—a poor orientation is likely to lead to turnover. Nurses learn in different ways, and the orientation should be individualized and results-focused. Part of the orientation should be in the classroom, with a unit-based component and self-directed learning modules, whether in the form of information packets, CD-ROMs, or web-based education.

New graduate orientation requires a very focused program that often is 12 weeks in length. For direct entry to a specialty unit, such as critical care or the operating room, orientation may be extended to six months. New graduate internships may also be offered that combine orientation, a consistent preceptor, classroom education in the specialty area, a low educator-to-staff ratio, learning goal assessment, support discussion groups, and self-directed learning modules. The culture must be supportive of new graduate RNs. If they are not mentored and supported, they will likely leave the organization within two years. The manager who allows new graduates to be treated poorly by experienced staff will never retain this valuable resource. Figure 7.2 provides a sample new graduate internship program for a tertiary teaching hospital in the Midwest.

Orientation programs must be designed to include some fun. To help new hires learn the names of staff, for example, create a crossword puzzle or word search with staff names included. This is a great icebreaker and a fun way for new staff to get to know other RNs.

Figure 7.2: Example of a Critical Care Internship Schedule

CRITICAL CARE INTERNSHIP
Summer 2002

Text: Hudak, C.M., et al. 1998. Critical Care Nursing: A Holistic Approach, 7th ed. Lippincott: Philadelphia, New York
All classes and clinicals begin at 0700. ALWAYS WEAR SCRUBS!

Date	MON	TUE	WED	THU	FRI
Week 1 July 1–5	System orientation AM: Asst. Clin. Mgr/CNS (16–19) • 16–17: Role of the CNS • Shift Report Content • Unit Chain of command/MD communication • Orientation binder, locker, etc.	Nursing Resource Center orientation Clinical Mgr. (16–19) • Rules of the road • Manager expectations	Nursing Resource Center orientation	HOLIDAY - OFF	AM : Asst. Clinical Manager/Infection Control (07–11) • Safety • Medication administration • Infection control PM : Respective Asst. Clinical Manager (1130–1530) • Introduction to patient care environment • Scavenger hunt • Unit tour
Week 2 July 8–12	Hospital orientation Reading: Chapters 15–20	System Critical Care Class (Cardiac A&P, ACS, CHF, Hemodynamics)	Nursing Resource Center orientation	Asst. Clinical Mgrs. (07–15) • CLINICAL patient assignment with the Asst. Clinical Mgr. • Focus on patient care environment	ACMs (07–15) • CLINICAL patient assignment with the Asst. Clinical Mgr. • Focus on patient care environment
Week 3 July 15–19	8° Reading: Chapters 22–26	System Critical Care Class (Pulmonary, mechanical ventilation)	8°	Care Coordinators (0700–0900) CV Care Managers (0900–1000) Cardiology Care Manager (1000–1100) Asst. Clinical Mgr.– Basic hemodynamic setup (1130–1300)– SICU CNS– Waveform analysis (1300–1500)– SICU	8°
Week 4 July 22–26	12° Reading: Chapters 5, 31–36, 43	System Critical Care Class (Neuro, Sedation, Diabetes, Pain)	12°	CNS– ABG interpretation (0700–0900)– CICU Resp. Mgr.– Ventilator Management (0900–1100)– Pulmonary 3E Asst. Clinical Mgr.– Review of Neuro exam (1130–1330)– SICU Asst. Clinical Mgr.– Review of Diabetic Protocol, Pain Scale, Palliative Care and Sedation orders (1330–1530)– CICU	12°

Week					
Week 5 July 29–August 2	12° *Reading:* Chapters 27–30, 37–40, 49	System Critical Care Class **(GI, shock, nutrition, renal)**	12°	Asst. Clinical Mgr– Fluid & electrolytes (0700–0800)– CICU Asst. Clinical Mgr.– Management of DIC (0800–0900)– CICU CNS– Management of shock (0900–1100)– CICU Nutritionist– Nutrition (1130–1330) CNS– Renal (1330–1530)– CICU	12°
Week 6 August 5–9	12° *Reading:* Chapters 7–8, 21 M/C interns switch sides	System Critical Care Class **(cv surgery, ethical, legal)**	12°	Skill Day	
Week 7 August 12–16	12°	NRC orientation	8°	12°	
Week 8 August 19–23	12°	Pharmacy (0700–1100) Unit Secretary (1130–1530)	12°		8°
Week 9 August 26–30	8°	12°	12°	Basic EKG	
Week 10 September 2–6	12°	12°		Basic EKG	12°
Week 11 September 9–13	8° NOCS	12°	8°		
Week 12 September 16–20	8°	12°	12°	With preceptor—Review of hemodynamic and pharmacology workbook (0700–0900)– CICU Final paperwork–(0900–1100)– CICU CNS—Care of the surgical patient (1130–1330)– SICU Asst. Clinical Mgr– 90 day evaluation (1330–1530)—Respective conference rooms	

Program developed by: Marinela Villejo, APN-CNS; Kathy Szumanski, MSN; Maria Barrionuevo, RN; Audrey Szczygiel, RN

Note: 8° and 12° are clinical shifts within the critical care units with an assigned preceptor and are not counted in nursing hours per patient day.

Source: Advocate HealthCare, Chicago, IL. Used with permission.

In-service Programs

In-service education is important to nursing staff, yet is challenging to provide in a meaningful way. Staff want and need information on new products, procedures, policies, and patient care; however, scheduling issues, time constraints, and the content itself may present barriers.

Motivating nurses to attend and learn from in-service offerings is also an ongoing challenge. A needs assessment should be done annually to identify the topics in which staff need training. To make in-service programs more appealing, those responsible for staff development may need to adjust the timing and structure of the training. For example, scheduling an in-service session at the change of shift is seldom effective. Nurses just ending their shift are probably tired and may have personal obligations to attend to. Nurses just coming on shift may be concerned about falling behind in their work. Instead, training should be held during the shift. "Learn at Lunch," an educational program with lunch provided; a poster session; small group in-service sessions; and train-the-trainer sessions, where one unit-based RN trains other staff, are very effective.

Educators should be creative with training. Different teaching methods can be adopted to accommodate staff flexibility and allow them to participate when their energy and interest levels are high. Educators might consider leaving audio- or videotaped lectures, handouts, and tests for staff members to take at their convenience. The educator should schedule a block of time when he or she will be available to answer any questions. Staff might also be provided with a self-learning packet containing theory and written procedures. A practice lab might be set up, in which nurses can stop in, practice a procedure, and take a quiz. Holding sessions on the clinical units is more effective than centralized education.

To keep nurses engaged, sessions should be interactive. Games can be used to liven them up. Structuring review content into games like bingo or Jeopardy helps nurses enjoy the session and remember the information. Role-playing can be fun for staff as well. Specific information can be distributed or posted; for example, the educator might post background readings on a new tool for pain assessment. A few days later, the educator can hold a session and ask a nurse to volunteer to be a patient in pain. Another volunteer can demonstrate proper pain assessment techniques.

Mandatory in-service training, such as that required annually by the Joint Commission on Accreditation of Healthcare Organizations, along with those the organization deems important, can be made interesting. Have various stations set up in an auditorium, with an educational topic covered at each station. Topics may include pain assessment, fire safety, infection control, bioterrorism, intravenous (IV) therapy, and so forth. Each station may have questions in a game show format, a word scramble, bingo, or other creative and interesting ways to help the RNs learn. Prizes can be offered to staff randomly or for accomplishing particular scores at each station.

Nursing Staff as Educators

In addition to using centralized education resources, wise managers will also use unit nursing staff. For example, if a nurse has been sent to an internal or external conference, that nurse can be asked to provide a brief summary at a staff meeting. This gives recognition to the growing knowledge of the nurse, helps to develop his or her communication skills, and updates other nurses on pertinent aspects of their practice.

Small, strategic assignments can be made to emphasize analytic and presentation skills. For example, a group of nurses can be asked to teach a workshop or design a training course for new hires. Nurses can be asked to develop a journal club, with the responsibility of identifying and distributing appropriate articles to their peers, leading discussion of the content, and implementing best practices from the reading.

Even errors can be used constructively to help staff grow educationally. For example, a nurse in a neurological/neurosurgical intensive care unit hangs the wrong concentration of sodium in the intravenous fluid. When the RN discovers and reports it, the nurse manager makes a unique request. Instead of chastising the RN, the manager asks her to research IV fluids and fluid and electrolyte balance and present an in-service session so the rest of the staff can benefit from the error. This nurse manager took a negative situation and allowed the RN and the rest of the staff to learn a valuable lesson. Error reporting should be encouraged. Consider using "good catches" instead of "near misses" as part of the nursing vocabulary.

Continuous Learning

When possible, send your best RN staff to trade shows and professional meetings. Encourage them to write presentations and publications. Also, tap the creativity of staff by asking them to issue press releases about unit successes, such as obtaining certain equipment or receiving a research grant. (Once written, seek the approval of your public relations department before release.) This exercise will allow nurses to help shape and craft the messages about their work environment.

When nurses come back from training sessions, they should be given assignments in which they can immediately put their training to use. Start with easy tasks and offer praise and feedback as soon as they have finished. You will see how effective the training was and help nurses to remember and put their new knowledge to work. Profile their accomplishments throughout the organization.

To create new challenges and learning experiences, assign nurses to small teams to accomplish specific objectives. For example, create a task force that visits a different unit to observe a known best practice, present an educational session at a middle school or high school, or recruit for nurses at a student fair. These activities require nurses to learn new tasks and deal with new people. Nurses may also be assigned to identify and address process improvement opportunities on their unit or another unit. This activity exposes nurses to process improvement or quality improvement opportunities and allows them to interact differently with peers.

Finally, continuous learning should not take place only in the clinical arena. Staff need education on a variety of interpersonal topics—conflict resolution, dealing with difficult people, time management, negotiation, communication, and other topics that will build the team and develop the staff.

Academic Positions

Work with a local college or university to obtain adjunct faculty appointments for qualified nurses. This serves to recognize the important work nurses do in mentoring and teaching nursing students and helps in the career development of practicing nurses. It also provides very real role models for nursing students.

In addition, schools of nursing can provide research opportunities for nurses who have such an interest. University faculty can be paired with interested nursing staff members to identify a research question, conduct a literature review, design and conduct a study, and analyze and communicate results. This can improve staff morale and contribute to the body of nursing knowledge.

CROSS-GENERATIONAL PROFESSIONAL DEVELOPMENT

Just as recruiting across the generations requires a variety of techniques, cross-generational retention strategies also must be tailored to meet different needs. Remember that one size does not fit all.

Use technology as frequently as possible for generation X and Net generation RNs. They expect to use technology and may be disappointed if the organization does not meet their needs. Ongoing professional development may be provided in a variety of technology-enabled formats, such as:

- interactive CDs that provide immediate feedback and are paced to the learner's needs
- Internet continuing education that includes content, testing, and certifications in certain specialties
- intranet continuing education that is developed within the organization on topics ranging from business conduct to mission and vision, from personal developmental to stress management
- closed-circuit television that staff can watch in the nurses' lounge
- audiotapes that can be listened to in the car, at home, or on the clinical unit on topics ranging from stress management to self-care

Many members of the latest generations to enter the workforce also want to use their nursing skills to help those less fortunate. Provide opportunities for volunteer work in charity care clinics, hospice organizations, perinatal outreach, and community endeavors such as health fairs, blood pressure screening, immunization programs, and accident prevention.

Listen to the professional needs of each generation. Employees need balance, opportunities for making an impact, and ongoing and continuous learning to stay loyal and committed to your organization.

MENTORING AND PRECEPTOR PROGRAMS

Preceptor and mentoring programs serve at least two purposes. First, they help retain nurses by appealing to their skills. Second, they help recruit nurses. Such programs are designed to honor nurses who exemplify high-quality nursing practice. They offer experienced nurses the opportunity to ensure consistent high-quality patient care. At the same time, they offer nursing students and new nurses a supportive and nurturing environment.

For the purpose of this chapter, preceptor programs are defined as carefully constructed experiences that pair an exemplary nurse with a nursing student. A mentoring program, on the other hand, is defined as a carefully constructed experience that pairs an experienced nurse with a new nurse.

Preceptors and mentors serve as coach and partner in professional and even personal growth. They inspire, guide, teach, challenge, recognize, encourage, and impart confidence. The relationship between preceptor and student and mentor and new nurse should be based on trust and open and honest communication.

Planning a Mentor Program

All new nurses need mentoring as part of their orientation. As with any program, planning is needed. First, management must agree that this is a necessary part of orientation. Next, the staff on the unit must identify what types of experiences should be included in the mentorship. This allows the staff to highlight how their unit may be different from other units in their organization. General objectives and a time line should be established. Ultimately, the experienced nurse and new nurse must agree on the specific goals to be accomplished.

Criteria for the nurse mentor must be established. Only nurses with excellent performance ratings who are interested in recruitment and retention should be involved. Excellent people skills are needed. Both full- and part-time RNs may be considered for preceptor and mentoring roles. The manager or director should approve any potential mentor. The following are characteristics to look for in the mentor:

- knowledge of self and others
- passion for work
- energy and creativity
- excellence in nursing practice
- commitment to caring standards
- ability to challenge and nurture
- honesty, integrity, and compassion
- ability to bring out the best in others
- openness to new ideas
- strong personal and business ethics
- commitment to improvements and lifelong learning
- appreciation for growth and accomplishments
- solid leadership skills
- willingness to commit to the program

Although mentoring opportunities are usually offered for new nurses, you may also want to develop them for experienced nurses who transfer into a new unit. Patricia Benner (1984), a nurse-author widely recognized as an expert on transitions in nursing, acknowledges that even expert nurses may become novices when practicing in new environments. You might even have a system in place that allows nurses interested in another unit to try it out with a mentor for a few weeks. Allowing nurses to move between units can help eliminate shortages during busy times and recruit new nurses into your unit. It will also help both the mentor and the nurse who is exploring the unit to stay challenged. Nurses can be paired for the time period or may shadow RNs in the new unit. A packet of information should be provided to assist the RN in understanding the new environment.

Planning a Preceptor Program

A tradition in nursing schools that is very helpful to students is to assign a "big sister." The big sister helps the nursing student survive nursing school by sharing strategies on how to study effectively, by listening to the student and showing empathy, and by providing support in challenging situations. Nursing students often feel uncomfortable sharing their innermost thoughts with an instructor, but will talk with a more senior student about concerns. Problems with an instructor, interpersonal issues with other classmates, or trepidation related to their ability to cope with terminal illnes or death and dying are topics that may be discussed with a student's big sister.

Today, most diploma schools have abandoned this tradition. As students in diploma, associate degree, and baccalaureate degree programs rotate to multiple clinical settings, they may not have the opportunity to bond closely with fellow students, faculty, or practicing nurses. Thus, the preceptor program was born.

A preceptor program allows a nurse to be paired with a student beyond the time when the student is doing a clinical rotation in the area of practice. The overall goal of the preceptor/student relationship is to support the individual as he or she makes the transition from student to nurse. Responsibilities of the preceptor and the student are clearly identified prior to initiating the contact. Sample preceptor responsibilities follow:

- Assume a leadership role in contacting the student and maintaining an ongoing relationship.
- Establish a relationship that is not intrusive and is comfortable for both parties.
- Once paired, remain in contact throughout the student's program of study, regardless of the location of clinical rotation.
- Mentor and coach the student by discussing academic issues, clinical issues, ethical and moral questions, and test anxiety.
- Make contact throughout the student's education program, especially during stressful situations—their first medication error, death of parent, failing exam, and so forth.
- Provide input on juggling a family life with educational and clinical requirements.

- Encourage the student to ask questions, seek advice, and discuss nursing issues.

As with a mentor program, a preceptor program involves planning. First, guidelines for the program must be determined. In particular, nursing administration must identify the aim of the program and estimate how many students should be accommodated. After the broad guidelines are established, the program should begin to recruit volunteer nurses. The characteristics to look for in a preceptor are the same as those given above for mentors. The characteristics and responsibilities of preceptors should be shared with the volunteer nurses, so they understand what attributes are valued. If a recruitment and retention committee exists at the institution, that group is in an ideal position to encourage and screen applications.

Recognizing Preceptors and Mentors

Preceptor and mentor recognition programs are often absent in the healthcare marketplace, yet are a key component of successful retention strategies. A number of strategies to reward preceptors and mentors may be used. Salaries may be increased by paying a premium hourly differential, for example. Scheduling preferences, such as a permanent shift, working fewer weekends, or working fewer holidays, may be arranged. Educational days may be provided to augment preceptor or mentor training and continuing education. Staff may be sent to a local education conference with a paid day off. A simple recognition strategy for a preceptor RN, for example, is to provide each with a preceptor pin he or she can wear on his or her name tag. An annual recognition event may be held. This might include the organization's executive staff to demonstrate the importance of the contribution made by these nurses. Small gifts or gift certificates might be provided. Whatever is planned, be certain to broadcast the event to as wide an audience as possible.

Evaluating the Programs

Both ongoing (formative) and outcome (substantive) evaluations are needed for preceptor and mentor programs. Frequent checkpoints should be implemented. Evaluation should not only be done at the end of the structured experience, but should be ongoing. A formal feedback system should be in place to identify and correct any program or learning-related deficiencies.

Evaluations should take into consideration the perspective of both the preceptor/mentor and the student/new nurse. For example, all parties can be asked to identify the positive aspects of the program and how to improve it. Preceptors and mentors should be asked what other tools they might need to mentor or precept more effectively.

In addition, other staff and management should have input into the overall evaluation. Of particular interest from an administrative perspective will be the tracking of new hires and their retention and accomplishments over time. In addition, the retention and career path of preceptors and mentors should also be examined.

GROW-YOUR-OWN PROFESSIONAL DEVELOPMENT PROGRAMS

"Grow your own" programs are an effective way to recruit into positions within your organization, and they can also be a very effective retention and professional growth strategy. The program enables staff to advance and grow without leaving the organization.

Nurses consider leaving their positions to take similar positions in their local healthcare markets for higher salaries, recruitment bonuses, and alternative scheduling. Some are moving into external nursing agencies for these advantages. Hospitals with declining profits find it difficult to provide sign-on bonuses, higher salaries than competitors, premium pay programs, or retention bonuses. They encounter problems with staff retention when forced to compete for nurses based on compensation alone. More importantly, money is a short-term solution, effective only until a competitor offers higher salaries. How can you compete?

The grow-your-own strategy is increasingly required to staff for the long term. Grow-your-own programming is generally targeted toward specialty areas, such as critical care, emergency department, labor and delivery, and operating room nursing. Identify hard-to-staff areas in your institution based on trends, and develop a program internally to cultivate your own specialty RNs, or collaborate with schools of nursing or community colleges. Several examples of grow-your-own programs are summarized in Figure 7.3.

Structured Learning

Both classroom and experiential learning must be provided in a grow-your-own program. Starting up such a program will occur more rapidly if curricula have already been developed internally or externally. Do not duplicate your efforts. Use learning devices and documentation that are already available and customize them to your environment. For example, the Association of Perioperative Registered Nurses offers educational programming that enables hospitals to grow their own perioperative RNs. View its web site, AORN .org, for further information (the course is available at AORN.org /education/perio101.htm).

Grow-Your-Own Programs for Students

Grow-your-own programs were mentioned as a recruitment strategy and can also be a career growth and development strategy for teens entering the workforce. This can be accomplished by collaborating with local high schools. The pathway begins prior to the senior year with a partnership between guidance counselors, leadership

Figure 7.3: Grow-Your-Own Programs for Specific Nursing Units

Current Area	Career Path Area	Requirement	Curriculum	Time (months)
Medical/ surgical	Adult critical care	One year of experience	• Self-study modules • Classroom lecture • Skills assessment/ development • On-the-job training	3–6
Pediatrics	NICU, PICU, or specialty pediatric units	One year of experience	• Self-study modules • Classroom lecture • Skills assessment/ development • On-the-job training • Rotations to each area	6–9
New graduate	Operating room	No experience	• AORN curriculum • Customized • Rotation to target services	6+
Psychiatry	Medical/ surgical	One year of experience	• Medical/surgical orientation • Skill building and assessment • Preceptor	3+

Note: NICU = neonatal intensive care unit; PICU = pediatric intensive care unit.

in the school, and the hospital or healthcare facility human resources department. Steps are outlined in Figure 7.4. This type of program is an ideal way for families with limited resources to afford college tuition and for potential students to develop a long-term career in your organization.

For example, if pediatric RNs are entering a formal program to transition into the neonatal intensive care unit (NICU), they would be assigned a mentor and either a nursing educator, an advanced

Figure 7.4: A Grow-Your-Own Program for Students

Time Frame	Path	Enablers
Junior year, high school	Students apply and are selected for healthcare track	Partnership with high school, human resources, and nursing; small class size (maximum 12)
Senior year, high school	Hospital education department provides assistance in education and training for students; trained as RN-assistive personnel	Curriculum designed by educational specialists and nurse educators; skills labs provided; instructors provided
High school graduation, age 18	Graduates apply for RN-assistive personnel positions; full- or part-time are selected	Open positions made available; supportive and timely human resources process assists students through the application process
Post–high school graduation	Students work full- or part-time with full tuition reimbursement for pursuit of nursing degree at local school	Tuition reimbursement; flexible schedule; supportive manager; assigned career coach
Two to four years post–high school graduation	Students graduate from nursing program and become full-time RNs	Publicity; open positions for new graduates; ongoing training and career development

practice RN from the NICU, or a unit-based NICU educator. An assessment of learning needs would be completed and an individualized education plan established for the transitioning RNs.

For the next six to nine months, the transitioning pediatric RN would attend classroom lectures, complete self-directed study, learn skills on the job in a structured setting in which he or she is paired at all times with the preceptor or unit-based RN, and rotate through various aspects of the NICU. He or she may start with more mature neonates or in a step-down area and progress into care of the most critically ill. Learning how to use monitors, ventilators, and pacemakers and performing technical skills are part of the structured learning. The goal is to develop confidence and the ability to safely care for the NICU patient population.

If your organization does not have available resources for student support, other options include scholarships or loan forgiveness. As part of the planning process, a number of these programs could be targeted. This is an ideal way to use the funding. Often, philanthropy can assist in this endeavor, and a number of grant opportunities also exist, especially for disadvantaged students.

This type of program is a significant commitment by the organization, but it pays big dividends. Be sure to structure agreements for this type of program to years of service in return for being a part of this career development strategy.

CAREER CONTINUUM RETRAINING STRATEGIES

The downsizing of nursing staff because of program elimination or difficult economic times in your facility or others in the area offers an ideal opportunity to build loyalty and retrain employees. Career retraining can be done through orientation, formal coursework, on-the-job training, and refresher courses. Nurses who have not been in the clinical setting for a number of years will need ongoing support as they develop their skills in a new area.

Nurses may choose to change their focus area or re-enter the workforce. The clinical area for refocusing or re-entry should be carefully selected to ensure success. Some key factors for success include the following:

- supportive culture and a manager who is willing to reorient and retrain RNs with a different skill set

- clinical support systems in place, such as advanced practice RNs and staff development
- nonspecialty environment for placement so the RN is not overwhelmed
- consistent mentor to help coach and support the RN
- ongoing, regularly scheduled continuing education with a focus on necessary skills to succeed at the new job

An illustration will prove helpful. A psychiatric RN with ten years of experience lost her job because the psychiatric unit was closed. She was offered a job in a medical/surgical geriatric unit. The RN needed a job but felt great trepidation in accepting the position. The staff and manager were welcoming. A staff educator from the nursing education department worked with her to develop basic medical/surgical skills. A seasoned mentor facilitated the RN's transition by supporting and coaching her during difficult times. After six months, the new medical/surgical RN felt comfortable in the new environment, and her education continued.

Nurses near the end of their career are ideal mentors and may work part-time or full-time in that capacity, without the physical demands of a heavy caseload and rotating shifts. Retention of new staff members is far more probable when seasoned preceptors help them learn a new skill set. A very talented, expert group of RNs training entry-level nurses is a winning strategy for both groups.

CULTIVATING A POSITIVE IMAGE FOR NURSING

Nurses have never been in a better position to take charge of their careers and influence working conditions. Raising the image of a career in nursing and promoting a positive image of nursing in the community is the responsibility of all nursing professionals. Instead of feeling tired, discouraged, and powerless, nurses need to focus on the valuable skills RNs bring to people's health and well-being. Nurses who feel good about their profession and their employer will stay in the profession and in the organization.

Speak Positively

A first step in cultivating a positive image is to continuously promote nursing. Help staff to recognize that the energy expended in denigrating the profession could be more positively focused. Support and encourage nurses to promote the profession in word and deed. Nurses and administration need to work together rather than argue about issues that divide them. They need to learn from each other. RNs need to fight for accessible, affordable, compassionate healthcare and for working conditions that make them excited about nursing. Speaking positively about the talents and skills of nurses; affirming coworkers, colleagues, subordinates, and supervisors; and recapturing the pride of being an RN will enhance retention.

When administration is respectful to nursing at every level of the organization, self-esteem is enhanced among the nursing staff. Administrative staff should openly and visibly promote the importance of nursing to the organization and speak positively about the significant contribution the RNs make. Positive patient letters about nursing should be read aloud at management meetings and published in newsletters.

Whenever the words, "I'm only the nurse," are heard, encourage the staff member to say, "I am *the* nurse." Being proud of the profession starts at the top and cascades throughout the organization.

Allow Input

Allow all nurses to provide input to senior nursing administration about their ideas, hopes, and dreams for nursing's future. These should not be gripe sessions but should provide an opportunity for staff nurses to voice their opinions. Management should welcome and appreciate ideas from staff nurses and others. Management will also appreciate ideas on how to improve working conditions and patient care. Forums include town hall meetings with the chief nurse executive and other senior nursing staff, e-mails to nursing administration, "sound-off" sheets that can be sent anonymously to the chief nurse executive, and so forth.

Identify Opportunities for Positive PR

Think of situations as opportunities for public relations efforts rather than problems. Opportunities have never been greater in the nursing profession. Nurses are in short supply and are being seen as a valuable resource rather than as a commodity. More than two million nurses practice in the United States, and RNs have tremendous credibility with the public. People think RNs act in their best interest, as nursing is one of the most trusted professions.

Leverage opportunities to increase nursing visibility. For example, nurses can appear on television and radio. Nurses have educated ideas and opinions that are valuable to the public. Call a local radio station or TV studio and ask if it would like to include a nurse as a regular guest to help listeners and viewers deal with the complexities of maintaining good health or managing access to healthcare. Perhaps your local newspaper would publish an "ask a nurse" column or print human interest stories about nurses and nursing. Nurses will feel more positive about their organization if it continuously promotes nursing.

An alternative is to join a speaker's bureau and be part of the local speaking circuit. Service organizations are always looking for speakers on a wide range of topics. Nursing experts who are interested and experienced in a particular topic can take it "on the road." Speaking to local groups will enlighten the public on the nursing shortage, the role it can play, and the challenges nurses face. Consider volunteering members of nursing administration to talk about nursing as a career at local schools. This exposes children to the profession and lets children know the great opportunities in nursing.

ENCOURAGING NURSES TO WRITE

Nurses have a powerful voice—encourage them to use it. A writing club can help novice writers get published. Provide information on the process of getting published and provide names, addresses, and web sites of nursing magazines and other avenues for publishing. An editorial may be a good way to get started. Seeing an RN's name in print is a powerful motivator, especially if he or she has been supported internally. Celebrate any type of publication your staff has been involved with—newsletters, staff forums, bulletin board reprints, and public recognition.

Nursing executives should also publish whenever possible. Showcase the innovations within the organization. Write a column in the local newspaper. Conduct interviews for nursing publications and the local press on any aspect of nursing that promotes and recognizes the profession and your staff. Nurses want to know they are well-represented and their accomplishments are recognized.

Finally, encourage staff to keep a personal journal and provide information to them to get them started. Writing or sharing personal reflections is helpful to many nurses.

SUMMARY

This chapter has covered a variety of topics related to career growth and professional development. Fostering self-assessment skills, developing an RN road map, and stimulating critical thinking skills all serve to promote lifelong learning. Educational opportunities for nursing staff may be provided in a variety of ways, including inservice training, using nursing staff as educators, continued outside learning, and academic appointments. Cross-generational professional development and orientation programs must be a part of the mix for career growth.

A variety of programs foster career growth and professional development. Mentoring and preceptor programs serve at least two purposes: they educate new nurses and students, and they enhance the professional development of staff. Mentor and preceptor programs must be carefully planned, implemented, and evaluated. Staff recognition for assuming new roles should also be included. Grow-your-own programs are effective for recruiting nurses for key specialties. They may also be used to recruit high school students into healthcare and nursing. Programs to retrain nurses are also needed.

Cultivating a positive image for nursing is an ongoing challenge in nursing and should be a focus. Encourage RNs to write, project a positive image, and utilize the media to identify nursing accomplishments and publicize human interest stories about nurses. Allow nurses to provide input.

REFERENCE

Benner, P. 1984. *From Novice to Expert: Excellence and Power in Clinical Nursing Practice*. Menlo Park, CA: Addison-Wesley Publishing Company.

CHAPTER 8

Reward and Recognition Strategies

INTRODUCTION

What is most important to practicing nurses? Recent research on nurses' job satisfaction suggests the two most important factors are evidence that what they do matters and stable and positive work relationships. Thus, reward and recognition programs must be not just gift-giving exercises, but instead recognize the important work of the nurse. The programs must be a reflection of how nurses are valued and respected by their managers and by the organization.

Managers play an important role in retaining nurses. The most important factor influencing an employee's decision to stay or leave is the kind of relationship existing between the nurse manager and his or her staff. Many staff nurses find their managers to be a greater source of stress than patients and families, other nurses, other healthcare professionals, and physicians.

Rewards and recognition contribute to a climate that fosters nursing satisfaction, and one can never provide too much of either.

IDENTIFYING POTENTIAL REWARDS AND TYPES OF RECOGNITION

It is very important to help managers appreciate the significant role they play in retention. Training managers as "chief retention officers" is very beneficial to the organization.

How do managers like to be recognized? What makes them feel valued? How might a nurse manager generate a list of rewards? One way to start is to ask the managers what motivates them. What could your boss do to demonstrate how much he or she values you? Give time off? A simple thank you? Something fun? Public recognition? A customized certificate? Knowing the answers to these questions is also very effective in developing reward and recognition efforts for staff.

For example, nurses may be asked what keeps them at the institution or in the department. A note card can be filled with the answers. Every month, the cards can be reviewed to ensure the RN has been recognized in a meaningful way. This provides the manager with a written reminder of what is important to the nurses and what you need to do so they remain on your team.

BUILDING AN INCENTIVE PROGRAM

Find Out What They Want by Asking Them

All good businesses have at least one incentive program. Regardless of the type of program, planning is key to its success. Incentive programs should be geared toward the needs of the staff. Have staff RNs help design the incentive program. Several steps may be followed to help ensure success when you develop an incentive program.

Identify the goal of the program. Start by clearly identifying the objective and stating the goal. For example, if the objective is to have nurses be more vigilant in identifying and treating pain, the goals related to that might be to provide faster response times to patient call lights, assess and manage pain using pain management protocols, or improve patient satisfaction regarding pain management. The goals must be measurable and as simple as possible. The more complicated, the more likely the efforts will fail. Also, the goals need to be fair and achievable for the entire nursing staff.

Select an implementation team. Appoint a team of nurses to obtain recommendations from their peers. Be sure to select a cross-section of nurses to serve on the team. Also make sure to have many views represented. After all, if everyone on the team agrees, there is no reason to have a team. Select people who will talk to their colleagues for additional views.

Select the reward or type of recognition. Charge the team with implementing goals. As part of this, the team should carefully identify the target audience. Programs driven by nurses themselves are the best and easiest to carry out. Be sure to encourage the teams to report to you any obstacles to improvements.

The teams should carefully consider the reward or type of recognition. The power of the reward or recognition is minimized if the nurse does not care about receiving it. The team needs to spend time talking about potential rewards and then select one that is within the identified budget. It may opt to provide several rewards and allow the winners to choose among them. Options may include extra time off, gift certificates, fewer rotations for a specified time, a close parking spot, a cleaning service, conferences or seminars, and certificates toward the purchase of uniforms.

Implement the program. Introduce the program to staff in brochures, staff meetings, unit posters, and one-to-one communication. Be specific about expectations and goals, time frames, and how the incentives are earned. If the staff achieves the goal, several options may be selected or one incentive agreed on, such as an extra day off biannually.

Market the program. Have your PR staff help with a brochure or flyer design and a "roll out" plan. Create a catchy slogan or name for the program to capture the nurses' attention. To roll out the plan, a kick-off event may be held in an auditorium or town hall meeting or by taking treats to each unit on a cart and handing out information.

Evaluate the program. Did the incentive program achieve its objectives? Were the nurses motivated to change their behavior? During the evaluation period, beginning to plan for the next incentive may be appropriate.

Remember that one size does not fit all. An effective motivation program today may not work tomorrow. Preferences change over time; do not be afraid to experiment. Ask your nurses what they like and be sure that staff are involved in organizing recognition efforts. To keep programs fresh, be open to trying new things. Evaluate what is working and what is not to learn from and expand your success.

REWARD AND RECOGNITION STRATEGIES

Low- and No-cost Strategies

Rewards and recognition need not be costly. In fact, no-cost or low-cost acknowledgments can be extremely successful. Nurses are motivated and have increased self-esteem when they are noticed and consulted. Acknowledgment of a job well done is grounded in respect and gratitude. Direct praise helps staff focus on self-esteem, self-respect, and recognition. A simple thank you expresses appreciation of the nurse's contributions.

Frequent Positive Verbal Feedback

One inexpensive way to reward and recognize nurses is to provide frequent positive verbal feedback. The feedback needs to be honest and include specific detail. Saying "You really kept your cool today when the physician was upset" is much more effective than "You do a good job." It is impossible to give too much feedback unless it is insincere. When you actually look for positive things, you will see them more clearly and help the rest of the nurses see them too. Praise nurses directly and also praise their actions to those who are important to them. This will reinforce the behavior you admire and build loyalty.

An example follows of how powerful a thank you can be. An RN made a comment to the chief nurse executive (CNE) in a staff meeting about how a high-risk obstetrician sought her out after working overtime during a high-risk delivery. He thanked her for staying—so simple, so powerful. The CNE mentioned it to the physician, and he was delighted to hear how much impact his simple thank you had on the nurse. He stressed to the CNE how appreciative he was of the nurse's skills and talents.

Written Feedback

Positive feedback may be given in a variety of ways. Managers can write down what they value most about each person, then communicate it. The note could say, "I really appreciate your great sense of humor when things get tough." A distinct notepaper color could be selected, and notes could be left for staff when they do good things. Nurses will begin to recognize the pattern and will look forward to being recognized in a positive way. Be sure to keep the notes positive. Otherwise, nurses will begin to dread receiving them.

For a more elaborate way of providing feedback, managers can create recognition business cards to give to a nurse after he or she completes a difficult project, achieves specific goals, or receives special recognition from a patient, family member, or physician. Managers could carry the cards with them to give out as the opportunity presents itself. A preprinted statement on the card can thank the nurse for his or her actions and suggest that the nurse bring the card to his or her next performance review. The manager writes on the card the nurse's name, the date, and the specific behavior being recognized.

To demonstrate support from nursing administration, consider creating a recognition memo on distinctive paper. The memo can be used as the recognition business card described above. Ideally, the chief nurse executive and all relevant department managers sign the recognition memo within 48 to 72 hours. If it takes two or three weeks to get the memo to the nurse, it is not a motivational tool. Rewards should be presented as close as possible to the good job that has been performed. For example, do not wait until the end of the month to recognize a nurse who did something special early in the month.

Prizes

Another option for an incentive program is to hand out small prizes. Managers could distribute "scratch and win" tickets when they see nurses doing something well. This is a fun and inexpensive way to reward nurses, and some may actually win a cash prize. Another morale builder used with success is the distribution of small discount coupons for ice cream. It is not the size of the prize that counts. In fact, having many small prizes is more effective than one large prize. Instead of a $50 gift certificate for a local store, consider giving five $10 shopping, movie, or restaurant certificates to five top nurses. This way, you avoid having one winner surrounded by upset and jealous losers who may have worked just as hard.

Making Rounds

Members of the executive staff should make rounds on the units or attend staff meetings periodically. Allowing nurses to see and be thanked directly by administrators fosters a sense of appreciation. Encourage administrators to gain a better understanding of nursing's contribution to healthcare by observing nurses firsthand.

While on rounds, consider taking pictures of staff doing their valuable work, and post them on a bulletin board in an area visited by patients and families. Include a short message about each photo, including the nurse's name. The nurse will appreciate the recognition.

Communication

Special accomplishments may also be communicated in institutional newsletters or even externally in nursing newspapers. For example, when a nurse completes a course or special certification, notify the public relations department and let them communicate to local newspapers and to any local nursing newsletters. (Often, specialty newsletters are published locally or regionally in areas such as critical care or rehabilitation nursing.) Alternatively, notify the community newspaper yourself to tell them about a nurse who attended a recent seminar or received certification. Consider establishing a "nurse of the month" award for your unit.

More Expensive Rewards and Recognition

Gift Certificates

If budget is not a problem, reward and recognition efforts may be designed on a grander scale. Gift certificates to restaurants, movies, sporting events, and other entertainment outings are always well-received. Employee luncheons and financial incentives can also be planned. Be sure to tie the rewards to excellent care. Otherwise, they will just be seen as a way to reward managers' favorites.

Celebrations

Parties can also be planned. This type of reward can help build a friendly, positive work atmosphere. Consider holding regular staff appreciation buffets, catered by managers and administration. Prize drawings can be included. Cookouts, picnics, or ice cream parties are easy to plan and let nurses know you appreciate the work they do. Of course, if the unit has 24-hour responsibilities, it is important to plan several get-togethers to allow all nurses to participate. Parties can be held at the unit level or throughout nursing.

A nursing recognition day can be planned to acknowledge the many contributions made by nurses. The goal would be to hold a one-day activity that would offer nurses an outing with friends and colleagues to network and socialize, enjoy refreshments, and demonstrate what makes nurses important to health and well-being. Corporate sponsors could be asked to provide services, such as massages, makeovers, and raffles for prizes. Schools of nursing could be asked to provide information on further education.

Remember, retaining staff is always cheaper than recruiting them. Recruiting, hiring, and training a new nurse can cost more than $20,000. Aim to keep your staff!

RECOGNITION FOR THE AVERAGE NURSE

When planning reward and recognition programs, do not ignore "average" nurses. These nurses, although often neglected, are important for reducing nurse turnover and improving work quality. Managers often pay attention to the performance extremes. Outstanding nurses make providing meaningful and specific feedback easy, and these nurses are more visible. Similarly, nurses who have performance problems come to the attention of management. However, providing recognition to your average nurse enhances care for the entire team and helps that nurse improve overall effectiveness.

All nurses need to know exactly what is expected of them. Nothing is more discouraging to staff than having to guess what their leaders want. Managers who offer only negative feedback on individual performance create doubt and confusion in their staff. Instead, let staff know how well they are meeting expectations. Ideally, positive reinforcement and recognition should be provided when things go right and constructive criticism offered when things go wrong.

Recognize and Motivate Average Performers

The manager can use a variety of techniques to recognize and motivate average performers. For example, the manager can describe an aspect of the nurse's performance that is above the standard and explain why it deserves special recognition. The manager should be specific about the performance and show positive emotion. He or she should explain why the behavior or characteristic is important to the unit. By praising a specific aspect of the nurse's performance, the nurse's confidence in his or her ability is reinforced.

In addition, the manager should express appreciation to the nurse for that behavior and indicate the desire to help in other aspects of performance. This demonstrates high interest in helping to develop the nurse's other capabilities and can be done by suggesting another area in which the nurse might excel. Specific steps or actions needed to enhance performance in a new area should be discussed. Suggestions should be solicited from the nurse and a plan developed between the RN and the manager. For example, an RN may have great interest in the care of the diabetic. The manager learns that the nurse has completed self-directed learning on the topic. The plan for building on the RN's skills and interests may include attendance at a conference, spending a day with the diabetes educator, and developing an in-service training session for the staff. The manager is showing confidence in the staff member and motivating her in an area of interest.

Maintain and Enhance Self-Esteem

When the manager addresses areas of average performance, it is important to maintain the self-esteem of the nurse and avoid the implication of a performance deficiency. The idea is to make a good performer even better, not give the impression that a problem exists. The manager should summarize the interaction and express confidence in the nurse. It is also important to have nurses recognize and appreciate each other. Small cards can be made and kept on the unit for staff to write in how another RN contributed or helped them.

SOLICITING NURSING INPUT AND BUILDING A RETENTION COUNCIL

Informal Interactions

Input from nurses can be solicited in many ways; never pass up the opportunity. For example, asking nurses what keeps them in their position or at your facility will reveal some interesting and important ideas. To uncover problem areas, ask some of the following questions:

- If you were king or queen for the day, what would you change about our unit?
- What could we do to retain you?
- If you had a wish list and could change anything about your job, what would it be?
- What should management do to make your job more productive? More satisfying?
- What new equipment or products do you wish we had?

In addition, managers can occasionally take a diverse group of nurses to lunch and ask them what they like and do not like about the unit or organization. Each shift may be taken out to breakfast or lunch every few months for an informal "gripe session" over pizza or pancakes. During the first hour, allow nurses to vent. Establish parameters for the venting: no personal attacks are allowed, no inappropriate or unprofessional comments or behavior are tolerated, and each complaint should be accompanied by a solution or recommendation. During the second hour, lead the staff in discussing solutions to the problems they have raised in the first hour.

Another effective technique is to ask, "What can your manager do more of or less of to help make this the best place to work?" Answers are very revealing and can be a springboard to action planning.

Appointing a retention council is an excellent way to solicit RN feedback in a formal way. Select RNs from across the organization who are informal, positive leaders with enthusiasm and creativity. Ask for volunteers. Provide ground rules for the group—are they advisory, or do they make decisions? Do they have a budget? Are they empowered to seek input from staff members, send out surveys, or conduct focus groups? By establishing the parameters and the reporting relationship in writing during the initial meeting, the council will rapidly develop retention ideas. It can also be empowered to develop its own rules and guidelines and present them to the administrative sponsor of the committee.

One small, rural hospital used this approach to tap the staff RN population to develop retention ideas. The staff committee recommended that marketing be done in a midsized city 20 miles away. An open house would be held to promote the merits of the family atmosphere, the financial stability, the excellent benefits, and the participative management style of the organization. The committee also recommended fewer rotations and a move toward permanent shifts by seniority and requested more flexible staffing alternatives such as part-time and 10- and 12-hour shifts.

Formal Mechanisms

At staff meetings, consistently put time on the agenda to discuss what nurses would change about the unit and how they would change it. Alternatively, hold a "recharge your batteries" contest. Ask nurses to suggest ways they can revitalize their jobs, then try to accommodate some of their ideas. Give an award to whoever comes up with the most creative proposal. During all interactions, encourage nurses to move beyond complaining about problems and toward solving them.

Another formal mechanism could be a morale committee. The committee may be unit specific or may extend across the organization. It is important to have diverse representation in the group. For example, the group should include nurses from every shift as well as nurses with various lengths of time in nursing and within the institution. An elected leader will help keep discussions on track. A morale committee helps provide nurses with a voice. The committee will give nurses the chance to identify concerns and ideas about their jobs. Most importantly, the committee can give suggestions for improving communications and retaining talented staff within the organization or unit.

Technology

Consider getting input via your company's intranet. Set up an e-mail address to allow nursing staff to post anonymous messages. Let everyone know that their input on what causes turnover and constructive ideas on how to decrease it is always welcome. This will allow you to identify potential policies, procedures, and problems that cause people to leave—before they leave.

INSPIRING NURSES

In addition to motivating staff, managers may also want to harness the power of inspiration. Motivation is an external force that pushes and prods us to get things done because consequences result if we do not. Inspiration is an inner drive that keeps us moving. It stirs our soul and stimulates our thinking. To shift from motivation to helping nurses tap their own inspiration, managers need to know their nursing staff, clear the path, and become a coach.

To know the nursing staff, spend time talking with each nurse about what assignments he or she wants to perform in his or her job. Why are they working? What excites them about their work? What accomplishments will make them feel successful at work? Once this is identified, it can be used to inspire them. Remind nurses how great they will feel when they accomplish something big for the right reasons. Find out what they really want and use it to inspire them.

To truly support nurses, eliminate everything that gets in the nurses' way of performing at a high level. As the manager, provide an environment that allows the staff to thrive. Get rid of useless paperwork, make sure they have the technology they need to succeed, set up flexible schedules, and involve staff in problem solving and interdisciplinary activities.

Becoming a coach is a necessary step in inspiring staff. When you are trying to inspire nurses to accomplish more and achieve at higher levels, remember they do eighty percent of the work. The manager needs to serve as the coach at the sidelines, helping the nurse win the game.

SUMMARY

Incentives are great for recognizing and motivating staff but should never be used as a bandage to solve unit problems. Incentives should complement monetary rewards and a positive practice environment, not replace them. Incentives must be deserved. If they are given to poor performers in the hopes of motivating improvement, they might send the wrong message that poor performance is acceptable.

Managers are very busy and may lose touch with the personal side of their job. However, they have the most immediate contact with nursing staff. As such, they are on the front line for verifying that what the nurse does matters and for fostering positive work and staff relationships. An insincere recognition and reward system will be quickly identified as such by nurses. However, a program that is put in place with the right philosophy will serve to motivate and retain nurses. Nurses will work hard to achieve goals that are reasonable and attainable.

This section has outlined key elements of a comprehensive retention strategy. Flexible schedules recruit and retain, as does encouraging work-life balance. Creating the right environment for the RN, one in which he or she has input, is respected and valued, and has a career that is nurtured, will contribute to the retention of the RN who wants a career in nursing. Monitoring turnover and intervening in problem areas are also essential for long-term success in nurse retention. Career growth and professional development are very important and should be fostered throughout the career continuum. All successful companies have reward and recognition programs.

This section concludes with Appendix 8.1, "Toolbox: 100 Ways to Retain RNs."

APPENDIX 8.1
TOOLBOX: 100 WAYS TO RETAIN RNS

Nurse Manager Retention Ideas

1. Ask each employee why he or she stays and keep the reasons on file. Check the file monthly to see if you have done your part in retaining the employee.
2. Hold workout sessions (open forums) to identify ways to improve the work environment. First, identify a topic for improvement, then generate ideas on how to improve, identify steps, set a date for implementation, and set a date for a follow-up session.
3. Write thank you notes by hand for employees to recognize their special contributions.
4. Seek feedback every day from your staff on how their work life could be improved.
5. Post a thank you Post-It™ note on the employee's locker.

6. Recognize employees in staff meetings, newsletters, and facility forums.

7. Call an employee into your office to thank him or her for something he or she did for patient care or the team.

8. Use one-minute praising frequently. Catch your employees doing something well and give them immediate and brief praise.

9. Never underestimate the power of on-the-spot recognition— for example, a pat on the back.

10. Create recognition cards. Encourage employees to give them to each other. Be creative with these cards. They may say a phrase that spells out "wow," "awesome," or any acronym you choose.

11. Post staff photos on a bulletin board on the clinical unit.

12. Keep small rewards ($5.00 value) and catch employees doing something right.

13. Write a personal note and attach it to the employee's paycheck.

14. Send an e-mail praising the employee.

15. Bake homemade treats for employees and hand deliver them.

16. Hold a departmental mini-retreat with staff; have managers and float RNs staff the unit during the retreat.

17. Write articles about employees for internal newsletters and local newspapers.

18. Have a departmental fun day and let the employees decide what it will be, as appropriate within the clinical setting.

19. Use certificates of recognition, tailored to the employee's contribution.

20. Provide departmental plaques for external or internal recognition.

21. Appoint RNs with excellent clinical skills as preceptors and provide rewards, a better schedule, or a differential.

22. Send birthday cards to your RNs at their home addresses.

23. Send a small floral arrangement to new RN hires to thank them for choosing you as their employer.

24. Buy the clinical unit something it wants—a toaster oven, new coffee machine, microwave oven, blender.
25. Put candy in staff mailboxes.
26. Pass out stress-relief kits to staff on an as-needed basis—include herbal tea, lotions, bubble bath, candles, etc.
27. Hand out "scratch and win" cards when you see staff doing great things.
28. Hold a unit potluck luncheon with the chief nurse executive, awarding prizes for the best food entry in several categories.
29. Initiate a "secret pal" exchange. Have staff members write on a slip of paper their name, birthday, and a short list of things they enjoy. Staff members pick one nurse's name, and the secret pal's mission is to do something creative and fun for the secret pal picked.
30. Provide a day off with pay and encourage the employee to use it for self-renewal.
31. Turn gripe sessions into opportunity sessions.
32. Never miss a chance to talk with staff about what motivates them.
33. Foster opportunities for senior management to interact with staff.
34. Hold a nursing contest to develop the best theme for Nurses' Week or hold a poster contest and select the best; award pizza parties to the winning units.
35. Establish a morale committee and implement at least five ideas.

Human Resources/Organizational Development Retention Ideas

36. Hold exit interviews with each employee.
37. Review exit interview data; identify trends and develop actions plans.
38. Ensure that each employee has the opportunity for professional development on the job.

39. Train first-line managers as chief retention officers.
40. Monitor turnover by department monthly. Hit the "stop" button if quarterly data show excessive turnover, and use retention improvement techniques. Identify issues with the staff that lead to turnover, and brainstorm ways to promote retention.
41. Provide scholarships for advanced degree completion.
42. Provide loan forgiveness programs—for example, forgive one year of loan payments for each year worked.
43. Hold nursing events for RNs and their families at a local amusement park or other venue.
44. Provide refer-a-friend bonuses.
45. Pay bonus or double pay to RNs who work extra hours, thereby avoiding agency expense.
46. Provide rewards based on years of service, and let employees choose from a menu of gifts.
47. Hold quarterly or annual years-of-service events.
48. Offer tuition reimbursement that is very competitive in the market.
49. Provide adoption assistance.
50. Provide subsidized child care with extended hours for the off-shifts.
51. Hold human resources–sponsored quarterly support groups for new graduates during their first year of employment.
52. Hold an employee or nursing talent show and provide work time for rehearsals.
53. Establish a career path for each RN.
54. Establish a student RN work/study program and offer tuition reimbursement.
55. Offer "care for the caregiver" sessions that teach staff how to reduce stress.
56. Promote nursing achievements such as degree completion, publishing, certifications, or special stories in organizational publications.

57. Teach RN staff, via in service training and case studies, how to diffuse angry people, including families, physicians, and patients.

Hospital and Nursing Leadership Retention Ideas

58. Establish a retention committee composed mostly of staff.
59. Provide a special parking place for employees who exemplify the values of the organization, and rotate the reward monthly.
60. Invite several staff members to have lunch with a senior executive or the CEO.
61. Have the chief nurse executive personally call or visit employees to thank them.
62. Send employees to a local specialty conference.
63. Start a recognition fund that may be supported through philanthropic or external grants.
64. Have the physician department chair or section director cook breakfast for the staff—a chef's hat and apron add to the festivities.
65. Hold quarterly or monthly town hall meetings.
66. Hold an employee picnic with prizes.
67. Deliver cookies and coffee or pizza to the clinical areas on very busy days when staff have difficulty finding time for lunch breaks.
68. Hold a ball in honor of nursing, funded by the medical staff.
69. Invite specialty nurses as guests of honor to the annual fund-raising benefit ball, the proceeds of which go to their department.
70. Invite staff employees to serve on facilitywide committees.
71. Ask your star RNs to consider promotional opportunities— do not wait for them to apply.
72. Provide free lunch coupons for managers to use for rewarding staff.

73. Provide recognition buttons for RNs for Nurses' Week.
74. Award gift certificates for movies, restaurants, book stores, and coffee shops based on a point system in which nurses can earn points for precepting, serving in the charge nurse role, committee work, extra hours, etc.
75. Provide career paths for RNs within your organization and train them in specialty areas.
76. Provide flexible work schedules that meet employees' lifestyle, such as 10- and 12-hour shifts, weekend programs, and night life programs.
77. Recognize your heroes and heroines in public places throughout the healthcare facility.
78. Reprint in the facility newsletter letters from patients or family members that praise RNs by name.
79. Provide exceptional employees with a mentor.
80. Enable employees to move into new positions.
81. Buy a tacky trophy and move it around the hospital for recognition purposes, such as best patient satisfaction, best associate satisfaction, etc.
82. Provide nursing sabbaticals; have RNs apply for a work sabbatical of up to two weeks. Select from applications that best meet criteria for improving patient care and will have an impact on improving nursing practice. The sabbatical could be used for nursing research, seminar attendance, a site visit to another facility, or gaining certification in a specialty.
83. Provide stress-relief baskets to managers with items such as relaxation tapes, body and bath items, herbal teas, stress-relief techniques; the chief nurse executive and senior leaders deliver them personally.
84. Have an ice cream social—with plenty of ice cream and toppings—and invite staff to come during their breaks.
85. Hold a holiday decorating contest and give prizes for the best holiday arrangement.
86. Provide nursing internships for new graduates and for RNs transitioning into a new area of specialty.

87. Create positions such as a sectionwide admission nurse (SWAN) to assist with the admission process between the emergency department and the units to decrease the burden on the nursing staff.
88. Use wireless technology to improve communication.
89. Develop a volunteer pool of recently retired RNs to serve in a counseling capacity by helping mentor, coach, and develop novice RNs.
90. Offer ethics consultations that can be accessed by RNs.
91. Offer critical incident stress debriefings for clinical units after a significant event.
92. Take care of your management team—take them off-site for an afternoon of relaxation and fun: choose among a variety of activities, such as a boat trip, cooking school, theater, luncheon, picnic, high tea, bowling, etc., based on your budget.
93. Offer excellent nursing students the opportunity to have a preceptor.
94. Bring a massage therapist to the unit to provide brief shoulder massages.
95. Provide a quiet, out-of-the-way "get away" room.
96. Identify, counsel, remediate, and remove if necessary poorly performing nurses.
97. Brag to the media about the good work nurses do.
98. Partner with a school of nursing to provide additional education and research opportunities.
99. Be sure the nursing staff is doing work only an RN has to do.
100. Create a blameless culture, by word and deed.

PART IV

Leadership and Management:
Strategies for Success

CHAPTER 9

Chief Nurse Executive: Role and Leadership Skills

INTRODUCTION

The role of the chief nurse executive (CNE) is a pivotal one in the organization and has evolved into a senior executive role. The CNE position usually requires an advanced degree, along with administrative experience and expertise in strategic planning, budgeting, human resources, and fiscal management. Often, the CNE attends board of directors meetings, medical staff executive meetings, and senior executive staff meetings. The right nursing climate is *created* by the CNE. The right nursing climate *retains* RNs. The right leader *develops* his or her competencies over time. A sucessful CNE must

- acquire emotional intelligence
- communicate a vision
- be visible
- prioritize
- incorporate leadership language

- listen
- provide feedback

The sections of this chapter discuss each of these aspects of being a successful chief nurse executive.

ROLE OF A CNE

Acquire Emotional Intelligence

What makes a chief nurse executive an exceptional leader, a leader RNs will follow, a leader who has a low nursing turnover? Nurse executives may have an advanced degree, impeccable professional and managerial skills, and seemingly the right experience to be a successful executive, yet when they reach the executive suite, they fail. Why? The answer may lie in the way organizations assess capabilities and develop their potential leaders (Kotter 1999).

As nursing leaders move into the executive suite, the presence of technical skill does not predict success. Intelligence, technical skills, and an impeccable resume of accomplishments are minimum requirements, but emotional intelligence (EI) is the differentiator between a good nurse leader and a great nurse leader. Emotional intelligence is described as "the capacity for recognizing our own feelings and those of others, for motivating ourselves, and for managing emotions well in ourselves and in our relationships" (Goleman 1998, 317–18).

Another attribute of exceptional leaders is emotional competence, which is learned and developed based on emotional intelligence (Goleman 1998). A CNE who successfully develops emotional competencies has a much greater chance of success in an executive role. Goleman's research has shown that EI is twice as important as intelligence and technical skills. EI serves as a predictor of employee performance; high EI accounts for more than 85 percent of exceptional performance in executive leaders.

The more complex the job, the more EI matters. Thus, the CNE must understand what these competencies are and how to develop the ones that matter. Why is this important to the CNE? Understanding and applying EI provides ideas on how to be a superstar CNE who will positively affect nursing and mold the staff into an aligned, high-performance nursing team. Good leaders can become exceptional leaders if they have the ability to manage their emotions and learn how to motivate those they lead. Motivated staff tend to stay with the organization, hence, emotional competence is an important concept to understand and develop.

Salovey and Mayer, in Goleman (1998), define emotional intelligence in terms of one's ability to self-regulate and self-monitor one's feelings and to use feelings as a guide for action. Goleman has adapted Salovey and Mayer's model to understand EI's importance in the work environment and has identified five components that determine a person's potential for learning skills: self-awareness, self-regulation, motivation, empathy, and social skills (Goleman 1998). Each component will be described and examples given to explain why these emotional competencies affect RN retention.

Self-Awareness

What is self-awareness? Leaders with self-awareness are confident, have insight into how their feelings affect themselves and others, know their strengths and limitations, and are aware of their biases. Self-awareness is a personal competency in which one knows oneself.

How does a leader develop this competency? CNEs with self-awareness know when they have offended their staff or managers by something they said or did. They know when they appear to staff as unfeeling or uncaring about their concerns or allow personal bias to interfere with their judgment.

Self-regulation

Self-regulation is the ability to control one's impulses and to channel moods constructively. Judgment is withheld until all facts are gathered.

The CNE who self-regulates considers major changes thoughtfully and presents them to staff in a rational, calm manner, considers all employee viewpoints, and will be trusted to be fair and non-judgmental.

The CNE who cannot self-regulate allows emotions and anxiety to overshadow positive traits. This is manifested in the CNE by angry e-mails or conversations, an accusatory tone of voice, and blaming, which create tension, anxiety, and upheaval among the staff.

Self-Motivation

Exceptional leaders are self-motivated and find great satisfaction in achievement, new challenges, and continuously stretching their capabilities. They are creative and energetic, and they seek new and better ways of doing things, often addressing problems without being asked.

CNEs with this trait are motivated to achieve success for its intrinsic value. That is, they seek success for the satisfaction of achieving success itself. A CNE may see a pending problem such as the closure of an area school of nursing and will proactively plan a partnership with staff and the school that keeps the school open and a steady supply of RNs for the institution.

Without self-motivation, the CNE is likely to be motivated extrinsically, that is, by such status measures as the title, the compensation, and the authority. Such a CNE spends most of his or her time building a power base, working only on projects that provide recognition and credit to him or her, and positioning for additional responsibility. The nursing staff's perception is that he or she is an advocate for himself or herself, but not for nursing.

Empathy

Empathy is a social competence and relates to handling relationships, a key skill in the CNE role. Empathy is the ability to consider and attempt to understand others' feelings, while still making sound decisions. This trait helps build trust, loyalty, and high-performing teams. Empathy is often associated with the nursing profession.

The CNE with this emotional competency can show concern for employees' feelings, while continuing to see the big picture. For example, staff may be very unhappy about a pay practice change and are expressing their frustrations to patients, physicians, and each other. Showing empathy for the feelings of staff, actively listening to them, and seeking open feedback helps build trust and loyalty.

A CNE without empathy might assert that things are "the way they are," a sentiment that allows no discussion or prospect for change, and will likely tell staff to look elsewhere for work if they do not like the situation. Listening to staff give meaningful feedback is not what this CNE does—and the staff act out as a result, often leaving the organization.

Social Skills

Social skills, the last of the social competencies discussed, involve managing relationships, building networks, collaborating, and communicating effectively. In exceptional CNEs, well-developed social skills are present, along with the abilities to influence, build teams, and lead.

This trait enables visionary leadership. That is, the CNE with excellent social skills inspires his or her staff, setting forth a vision for the unit or organization as being the premier place for professional nursing, and articulates what that means. Staff come to understand that the CNE is a nurse advocate, seeks to advance the profession, and recognizes and appreciates nurses of all levels. He or she meets with staff at all levels and on all shifts and builds constituencies with the public relations, finance, human resources, and marketing departments to make the vision a reality. Staff believe this is possible because of his or her presence.

Without this key trait, the CNE will flounder. The level of performance of the nursing staff will stagnate, and turnover will be high. This is a CNE who cannot relate to staff. For example, in one hospital, when a difficult staffing change was made, the CNE attempted to talk to staff, but because of an absence of social skills, she was seen as defensive and unsupportive. This reaction resulted in a major campaign to unionize the nurses, polarizing staff and management. In the end, the CNE was replaced.

High EI quotients are becoming increasingly important in executive and senior nursing leadership because organizations are now facing rapid change, mergers, downsizing, and restructuring. The CNE with high EI will lead employees by sharing a common vision, allowing time for the fundamental changes to be absorbed. Employees and managers need leaders with high EI—which can be developed into emotional competence—to not only survive, but also thrive.

The CNE who will struggle with his or her role is the one who has a low level of emotional competence and who thinks employees should be grateful to have a job. He or she labels staff as troublemakers or resisters and reacts to problem situation accordingly, further inflaming them. A CNE without these skills who terminates a manager or director may be sending the message that "it is my way or the highway."

Most organizations cannot afford a CNE with low EI for very long. Staff will indicate their displeasure by leaving the organization.

How can a CNE build EI and develop emotional competencies over time that will enable him or her to recruit and retain staff?

1. Self-awareness
   - Use 360-degree feedback from your staff and colleagues to validate how aware you really are of issues, challenges, and obstacles identified by your staff. This method of feedback is a process in which direct reports and colleagues provide structured, written feedback to you or your boss about your strengths and growth needs.
   - Know your biases and reserve comment when an emotionally laden topic is discussed by the staff.
   - Ask others you trust to critique you and point out behavior that you do not recognize as harmful to staff perceptions.
2. Self-regulation
   - Never jump to conclusions or make hasty judgments—always hear all sides of a story before reacting.
   - Think before you act—if it would feel really great to make a statement, you probably should not.
   - Always be honest and straightforward with your staff.
   - When challenged, remember the basic skill of listening—do not react.
   - Be open to innovation and new ideas identified by your staff and managers.
3. Motivation
   - Seek out challenges and volunteer to take them on for the organization, especially if they will have a positive impact on nursing.
   - Proactively address nursing issues before they become problems.
   - Follow your passion for achievement in areas that matter to you. Do what you love.
   - Mentor and coach staff—train your replacement.

- Show your optimism, bounce back from obstacles, and persevere in your goals.
4. Empathy
   - Deal directly with resistors, be they staff or managers, and listen to their reasons; try to understand their perspective on volatile issues.
   - Watch for cues of dissatisfaction, distrust, and unhappiness and address them by using "I" messages. For example, rather than confronting a situation directly with the comment, "You are so negative and unhappy that people avoid you," the CNE could use an "I" statement: "I am concerned that you seem so unhappy. What can we do to improve the situation?"
   - Avoid taking on the parental role, taking sides, or trying to convince others your position is correct.
   - Coach and mentor—provide ongoing, honest feedback to your managers and staff.
   - Do not become involved in the personal lives of your managers or staff or develop friendships that are too close for you to remain objective.
5. Social Skills
   - Work on conversational skills—engage staff whenever possible.
   - Take courses in public speaking, negotiation, and persuasion—build on your skill set.
   - Engage many different and diverse audiences on controversial topics and facilitate their discussion
   - Inspire your team—set the vision.
   - Practice "high touch" with your staff with frequent interactions at staff meetings, coffees, and open forums and while walking around the unit. That is, be present, be available. Do not just be accessible on the telephone or by e-mail.
   - Study change techniques; be a master change agent.

By enhancing your emotional intelligence, you will be a leader who enjoys staff respect and trust—a leader to whom staff" are drawn, a leader who has created a high-performing nursing team, and a leader for whom staff want to work.

Communicate a Vision

It is important to develop a nursing vision. It motivates and inspires staff and sets a common direction for all to follow.

The hospital usually establishes its mission, vision, and values. The mission and vision may change as times change, but values remain constant. The CNE may in turn establish a nursing mission, vision, and set of values or may choose to adopt hospital mission and values and create the nursing vision. Ideally, the nursing mission flows from and is consistent with the overall organization's mission.

The mission statement describes the overall purpose of the organization—why does it exist? Within nursing, the question is, "why does it exist at this hospital—to do what?" Figure 9.1 provides a sample nursing mission.

Values represent the organization's core priorities, or how employees are expected to act. Accepted values may include caring, compassion, stewardship, excellence, teamwork, continuous improvement, and other words that reflect how employees are expected to live out the mission of the organization. These core values usually reflect those of the hospital and of the nursing profession.

Establishing a vision statement is important to nursing: If you do not know where you are going, any road will get you there. To establish the direction or vision for nursing, the CNE and senior management team must develop the vision and communicate it to every corner of the organization. Nurses will embrace something that is meaningful to them and take pride in what nursing contributes.

Figure 9.1: Advocate Lutheran General Hospital's Nursing Mission

Nursing is both an art and a science, responding to the human condition. The nurse-patient interaction involves the whole person, focusing on body, mind and spirit. Nursing interventions are designed to promote the patient's physical, mental, and spiritual health.

Grounded in the nursing process, nurses assess, analyze, plan, implement, and evaluate care based on the needs of the patient. While nurses may delegate aspects of care delivery, the professional nurse possesses the critical thinking skills necessary to lead the patient care team.

Nursing is an interdependent practice, requiring collaboration with patients and other health care providers. The five Advocate Health Care values (compassion, equality, excellence, partnership, and stewardship) serve as an internal compass to guide nursing relationships and actions.

Continuous quality improvement and nursing standards of practice are the foundations for nursing quality; both are critical to the achievement of optimal patient outcomes.

Research and its application are necessary for the development and enhancement of the nursing profession. Ongoing education is essential for the development and maintenance of competent nurses.

Source: Advocate Lutheran General Hospital, Park Ridge, Illinois. Used with permission.

What Is a Nursing Vision?

A nursing vision is a target that beckons staff—a mental picture of what the unit, department, division, or organization can become. A good vision is futuristic and compelling.

Why does nursing need a vision? The vision sets a tangible direction and centers around a common desire to improve. It captures the attention of your staff as it articulates for them the dream of being better. It answers the question, "what can we be?"

Figure 9.2: Examples of Nursing Vision Statements

Clinic Nurses—Des Moines University Clinic Nursing Vision Statement

We are recognized as Ambulatory Care Nursing Leaders in a progressive environment where we improve the health and wellness of individuals, groups, businesses and communities.

Geisinger Health System Vision Statement

To be recognized as a leader in nursing practice and the nursing career provider of choice.

Sources: Used with permission of Des Moines University Clinic, Des Moines, Iowa; and Geisinger Health System, Danville, Pennsylvania; respectively.

How Is a Vision Developed?

You can be highly analytical and research vision statements of other nursing departments, complement your hospital's vision with similar concepts, or use focused discussion, brainstorming, or storytelling to capture concepts. Involve as many nursing leaders and staff as possible—get feedback on draft statements from different constituencies. The vision needs to be compelling—if it is not, return to the drawing board. A compelling vision is one that has meaning for the nurses; it must resonate with them and describe what they want to see in nursing. Figure 9.2 provides two examples of vision statements.

True nursing leaders inspire commitment to the vision by speaking the language of nursing and by understanding nurses' dreams, needs, and interests. True leaders also show great enthusiasm for the vision. Leaders use "we" and enlist the support and assistance of all levels of nursing. Teamwork, trust, and empowerment of staff turn the vision into reality.

Be Visible

To lead and build credibility within the nursing organization, the CNE must be visible and demonstrate that he or she cares about nurses. Effective CNEs lead by example and model what they expect from the administrative team. They support nursing and are continuously trying to improve every aspect of the nursing division. They are visible to the staff by making rounds on the clinical units, holding town hall meetings, attending staff meetings, being a spokesperson for nursing, recognizing staff in many different ways, sending handwritten notes, and involving staff in the business of nursing at all levels. Being on the forefront of innovation is a critical success factor; networking, reviewing the nursing and healthcare literature, participating in seminars and conferences, and learning in self-directed programs keep the CNE abreast of trends and on the cutting edge of effective leadership.

Leading effectively also requires continuous feedback through staff satisfaction surveys, focus groups, staff meetings, workout sessions (open forums) on targeted topics, and other means—all designed to identify what nurses want and need, and how needs can be met.

CNE LEADERSHIP SKILLS

Characteristics of admired leaders are described in Kouzes and Posner's (1993) book, *Credibility*. Frequently mentioned behaviors include the following:

- is supportive of staff
- has the courage to do the right thing

- challenges staff
- develops others and acts as mentor to others
- listens
- celebrates accomplishments
- keeps commitments and follows through
- trusts people
- empowers others
- makes time for staff
- shares the staff's vision
- has an open-door policy, in which staff are encouraged to consult the manager at any time
- overcomes personal hardships
- is able to admit mistakes
- advises others
- is a creative problem solver
- is a good teacher and coach

This list of behavioral dimensions centers on the staff and on developing them, listening to them, empowering them, and making them feel important. It is not about the importance of being the CNE.

Leading is about mobilizing others to want to go in the same direction—great leaders challenge, inspire, motivate, empower, enable, and serve as a role model and coach. Staff will perform for a merit raise, for a promotion, to stay employed, and for other extrinsic rewards. However, leaders enlist support and gain commitment because staff believe in them; staff will perform at a higher level when they are motivated by intrinsic rewards—knowing they are doing the right thing, job satisfaction, and knowing the good work they do is acknowledged and appreciated—that come from belief in a leader and an organization.

Leaders who are able to tap the heart and soul of the nursing staff will have organizations that are worlds apart from those that are headed up by leaders who stay only because of the weekly paycheck.

Managing Your Leadership Skills

Staff need and want an exceptional leader, a leader they see often and with whom they interact. The CNE wants to be the best possible leader and at the same time has many priorities, such as meetings, budgets, personnel issues, strategic plans, and staffing challenges that are ever present. There are not enough hours in the day to be visible, to talk to staff, to seek feedback, or to recognize and reward.

How can all this be accomplished—having the important soft skills when the hard skills take most of the CNE's time and energy? Soft skills retain staff, yet hard skills are needed to manage the business of nursing. Many ways exist to balance both the hard and soft skills that make a CNE successful. The sections that follow characterize some of these ways.

Prioritize

CNEs must learn to prioritize their time using effective time management skills, delegating, and balancing organizational needs and nursing needs. The executive calendar is a good place to start; to increase chances for success, the usual routine must be altered.

First, all "must attend" meetings must be left on the calendar. With all other items removed, work with your secretary to re-evaluate your appointment organizer and begin to fill in the calendar and create your new routine. Build in walking-around time each week. Schedule quarterly town hall meetings on your calendar. Identify several off shifts you can visit, and block out the next day for these visits. Set up time to attend one staff meeting per year for each unit. Screen every meeting and ask if it adds value to your role as a leader. Screen all requests for meeting time. Delegate tasks and handle some situations by phone or electronic mail instead of in person to free up time for nurses. Learn to say "no."

Delegation is an important skill, and it helps managers and staff grow professionally. Delegating tasks and projects to work groups of staff or managers enables them to add variety to their jobs and develop skills. Good examples of tasks that should be delegated to a senior nursing leader, with staff involvement, include designing a self-scheduling program, helping in nurse retention efforts, planning activities for Nurses' Week, designing documentation flow sheets, participating in continuous quality improvement activities, and enabling nursing staff.

Staff who are appointed to committees feel recognized by senior leadership. Use your RN talent; it abounds in the organization.

Incorporate Leadership Language

Talk to staff often. This makes a difference. Rather than being viewed as an ivory tower executive, a CNE who has contact with staff appears human and approachable. Use words and phrases that inspire and motivate your staff, and use them often to build loyalty and commitment in your organization.

1. "You did a great job on this." Give positive feedback to managers and staff on a job well done.
2. "I made a mistake." Apologize and acknowledge when you have made a mistake or a poor decision. Talk about why your action or decision did not work and what you learned. Use your error as a tool to move toward a blameless culture.
3. "We are a strong team and can get this done." Use this phrase for challenging situations and crisis periods. Let everyone know you are all in it together. Overcommunicate.
4. "How do you think we should do this?" Ask managers and staff for their opinions and ideas, as they are your best resources. Listen carefully to the answers and incorporate them as appropriate. Provide public credit for the ideas.

5. "Let's look at another way to accomplish this." When managers and staff are going down the wrong path, provide alternatives and walk them through the positive and negative consequences of each.
6. "I don't know the answer but will find out." Do not be afraid to say you do not know, and always get back to staff when you get the answer.
7. "I want to get more information in order to really understand this situation." Do not make snap decisions based on one version of a story or conflict. Investigate and get the facts. Talk to all involved parties. The truth is usually somewhere between various versions of what happened.
8. "I want you to lead this effort for me. I know you will be successful." Stretch your staff. Give them challenging assignments and mentor them through those assignments. Praise them when the assignments are completed.
9. "Let's look at how we can improve next time." This is particularly important when mistakes affecting patient care have been made. A blameless culture is the ultimate goal.
10. "How am I doing?" Seek feedback on your performance on an ongoing basis. Ask how you can do better. Do this verbally or seek written feedback. Ask, "What can I do more of?" and "What should I do less of?"

Listen

A common complaint within nursing is the nurses' lack of voice in organizational decisions affecting them. This can lead to low morale, turnover, and dysfunctional behavior. The CNE's words and deeds, more than with any other nursing leadership role, affect whether the nursing staff feels its opinions and needs are taken into consideration.

Walking on rounds several times a week and holding individual conversations with staff is a simple yet powerful strategy. Ensure that your leadership team does the same. Hold nursing forums by section (critical care, pediatrics, medical/surgical), at the nursing clinical unit, or for the overall nursing division several times a year.

Each year, invite nursing staff to hear you outline the vision and goals for the upcoming year, as well as industry trends and challenges. Provide an open forum for questions, either written or verbal. Acknowledge each and provide honest and straightforward answers.

Involve your management staff in decision making. Carefully identify those types of decisions that the senior executive nursing team must make, and identify those that can be delegated to the middle-management group. Delegate as many decisions to this key group as you can, especially those that affect their role and their staff. When developing new programs, have nursing managers involved; they will have input that the senior team will not.

The voice of the staff RN can be elicited in many ways. These include the following:

- Establish a facilitywide clinical practice council with a representative from each area.
- Establish a clinical excellence council at the unit level to focus on patient care delivery improvements.
- Attend staff meetings and seek input on a variety of nursing-related issues.
- Appoint staff RNs to facilitywide committees related to issues affecting their practice.
- Involve nursing staff in solutions to challenging issues such as cost reductions, sentinel events, or programmatic changes.
- Share information with staff, both positive and negative, and allow honest reaction and feedback.
- Provide an anonymous forum for staff to be heard—through the Internet, a mailbox in a central nursing location, or by way of the human resources department.
- Encourage the development of a nursing-staff or unit-based newsletter written by staff.

- Listen to the new graduate voice. Hold quarterly support groups and assist in the transition to actual nursing practice.
- Provide choice to staff. Self-scheduling is one way to give RNs a voice in work-life balance.
- Conduct RN associate surveys at least annually and provide feedback at the staff level.

Provide Feedback

Staff members can never get too much feedback or too much praise. The norm, however, is to provide very little or none at all. Encourage a continuous feedback loop from your senior leadership team. Make public any complimentary patient letters about staff members by publishing them in facility newsletters or posting them in prominent locations. Tell stories about your heroes and heroines. Send stories to the local newspaper. Encourage managers to say "thank you" after an extra shift or a difficult situation, post notes on RN lockers praising their accomplishments, and pick a nurse of the month.

Letters or notes from the CNE thanking or acknowledging staff are very powerful. For example, a note may be written to a nursing educator thanking her for the superb educational event he or she developed on pain management. A note to a staff RN who went above and beyond expectations for a patient's family is very much appreciated and will be widely discussed. Even in negative situations, such as sentinel events, it is important to praise staff for being willing to talk about the event and learn from it. An open CNE who accepts feedback, seeks feedback, and encourages feedback is the CNE for whom most RNs want to work.

Feedback from satisfaction surveys, focus groups, or interviews should be provided to the staff in a timely manner. Show the positive and the negative responses. Address problematic areas and ask for solutions and ideas. If you are not willing to provide feedback, do not conduct the surveys or staff interviews.

It is also important to provide feedback to the medical staff about nursing. Keep them abreast of challenges and issues. Medical staff leadership and physicians can be a powerful force in helping RNs feel positive about their practice by acknowledging their efforts and issues and by validating their role as peers. Address physician behavioral issues with the chief of staff or directly; policies should be in place to promote zero tolerance for inappropriate physician behavior. Allowing behavior such as verbal harassment, inappropriate conduct, yelling, belittling, and so forth, is a sure way to cause staff turnover.

SUMMARY

The CNE role is pivotal to retention in any healthcare organization. Although hard skills, such as budgetary management, personnel management, and strategic planning, are important, emotional competencies are equally as important, or more important. Developing emotional competencies will enhance the CNE's leadership abilities and ensure staff remain loyal and committed to the organization. Emotional intelligence and its role were discussed.

Leading the organization requires developing and articulating the vision of nursing and putting forth the dream of what nursing can be. Several sample vision statements were provided, and ways to lead the organization were identified. The CNE sets the tone for what nursing is, how nursing is viewed, how nursing acts, and how nursing is valued. Most importantly, because of the CNE, staff see what nursing can be. Staff want to be a part of the organization the CNE has created. Staff will stay in this type of organization.

Ways to ensure that the voice of nursing is heard and enhancing participation in decision making concluded this chapter. Leadership is all about getting extraordinary things done. Senior leader and manager roles are also a critical success factor and will be discussed in Chapter 10. Without followers, a leader has no one to lead.

REFERENCES

Goleman, D. 1998. *Working with Emotional Intelligence*, Appendix 1. New York: Bantam Books.

Kotter, J. 1999. *What Leaders Really Do*. Boston: Harvard Business School Press.

Kouzes, J., and Posner, B. 1993. *Credibility*, p. 50. San Francisco: Jossey-Bass.

Role of the Senior and Middle Nurse Manager

INTRODUCTION

Decisions related to the promotion of personnel within nursing are very important, because the right management team is necessary to create an exceptional work environment. Such an environment is one that motivates, retains, inspires, and fulfills its nursing staff and builds a loyal and committed RN workforce. Traditionally, nursing promotes from within its ranks, from manager to director, from the best clinical nurse to manager. Although this method of promotion may be successful, at times it fails. Why?

Required competencies change as a nurse enters the management arena. The newly promoted manager may not succeed long term without fundamental competencies needed in management and leadership roles or without professional development and coaching. Interpersonal skills become more important; technical skills lessen in importance.

This chapter focuses on what is required to be a successful nurse manager and provides strategies for senior nursing leadership and middle managers.

ROLE OF THE SENIOR NURSING LEADER

In a healthcare hierarchy, having a level of management between the senior executive and the middle manager is common. Titles vary, but those frequently used are director, clinical director, and assistant administrator. Often, this level of management provides a promotional opportunity from a middle manager position. Organizationally, depending on the size of the facility, the senior nurse leader (SNL) may oversee sections of nursing areas such as critical care, women's health, and medical/surgical.

Given the complexities of healthcare organizations, the chief nurse executive (CNE) must depend on his or her administrative team to be the eyes and ears of the nursing segment of the organization. Effective SNLs manage large portfolios (i.e., they have many responsibilities in various venues) and address issues and problems on a daily basis. A senior leader who is available to staff gives the nurses an administrative link that can facilitate solving the problems and answering the questions on a day-to-day basis that their direct manager may not be able to handle.

Senior nurse leaders mentor and coach their first-line managers, who act as the chief retention officers within nursing. Managers who feel supported will in turn be able to support their staff members.

Competencies of the SNL

Technical skill is not a requirement within the SNL role. Although understanding the clinical environment is beneficial, the SNL often oversees a broad portfolio of clinical departments, and strong technical skills will not likely be present in every SNL of every area. Technical skills *are* often a success factor at the middle nurse manager level, so the SNL can rely on the expertise of the middle nurse manger for assessing clinical situations and the technical skills of RN staff. The SNL usually holds a master's degree.

Competencies needed in the SNL mirror many of those that ensure success in the CNE role. Emotional intelligence is important and should be developed and enhanced within this role. Important competencies include the following:

- Excellent interpersonal skills
- Ability to communicate effectively
- Ability to build teams and partnerships
- Broad critical thinking skills
- Negotiation and conflict resolution skills
- Ability to think creatively and innovatively
- Ability to work well with physician leaders

This role ensures that the vision of nursing is known and understood by managers and staff. The SNL may be a very visible, hands-on position or may be more administrative, with a focus on budgets, planning, or project management. A hybrid role definition is also possible.

From the staff RN perspective, the most credible leaders are those they know. Thus, the highly visible SNL who makes rounds on the clinical units, is actively engaged in initiatives, knows staff by name, is actively engaged in the business of nursing as a champion, and is the voice of staff to senior leadership will enjoy more respect and trust from the staff.

A balance between administrative responsibilities and soft skills is challenging, but can be managed. Ongoing professional development builds competencies and skill and leads to career fulfillment and promotional opportunities.

To be the best SNL, ongoing growth and development can occur in multiple ways:

- Find a great mentor.
- Attend advanced education courses or targeted classes in spreadsheet applications, business planning, finance, and so forth.

- Join professional organizations.
- Use the Internet for self-directed continuing education.
- Attend national conferences.
- Network with others in your position.
- Seek 360-degree feedback and build on constructive criticism
- Volunteer for tasks that stretch your skill base, such as new or temporary job assignments, task forces, or special projects.

HOW CAN THE SNL LEAD EFFECTIVELY?

SNLs can motivate and inspire their staff members by promoting an environment that fosters teamwork, collaboration, innovation, and passion for what they do.

1. *Build loyalty:* Praising employees by complimenting, congratulating, and commending them in public or private forums or using other forms of recognition by way of newsletters, pictures, stories, and public exposure to showcase your staff builds loyalty.
2. *Build commitment:* Fostering a climate of excitement, enthusiasm, and innovation in which your staff are very involved builds commitment.
3. *Retain staff:* Creating a high participation environment in which each staff member feels he or she has a voice in issues of importance to them retains staff.
4. *Be available:* Availability is very important to staff and managers. Middle managers as well as staff need SNL support, including having the SNL available for them when needed. SNLs should give middle managers the skills and coach them on how to be a great manager, but should not be doing their jobs for them.

What Middle Managers Need from the SNL

Middle managers in all industries experience the feeling of being uninformed and not a part of what is happening. They may feel like they are the last to know about developments or decisions. This situation is not ideal. snls depend on rn middle managers to coordinate the activities of very complex operating units. Supporting middle managers requires focus and consistency. A number of practical management strategies can be used by the snl that will help create an effective working relationship:

- Be very clear on the expectations of the role of the middle manager and the expected results; interact frequently and ask for periodic updates.
- Provide coaching and professional development opportunities whenever feasible; offer ongoing professional development through internal and external courses, seminars, personal development plans, and self-directed learning.
- Provide ongoing feedback on performance that is both constructive and includes recognition and praise for contributions.
- Listen: ask for ideas, feedback, and opinions and bounce ideas off middle managers.
- Support middle managers in work-life balance.
- When middle managers face difficult staff, challenging physicians, and crisis situations, be present and available.
- Hold middle managers accountable; be specific on what that means.
- Delegate if the manager is ready for additional responsibilities; be sure the manager does not feel that he or she is doing the snl's job.
- Prepare managers for the next step. Can they become the snl? If so, develop them for the role.

ROLE OF THE MIDDLE NURSE MANAGER

The role of a middle nurse manager (MNM) is complex and challenging, one in which many priorities must be juggled. In recent years, the role has been identified as critically important in staff retention. Staff usually do not leave organizations, they leave their bosses. The MNM is the leader closest to the staff role and thus is in the best position to monitor staff satisfaction. In addition to retention, the MNM is responsible for overseeing patient care delivery, monitoring quality assurance and improvement, and managing a large RN and support staff workforce with the multiple personnel issues.

Skills Needed for Promotion

Healthcare organizations commonly promote to middle management the best staff RNs who show clinical expertise and leadership potential. However, skills learned in nursing practice may not prove to be the skills needed most in a managerial role. Within nursing practice, skills are learned through formal education and continuing clinical education. Positions in management, on the other hand, focus more on people skills, which managers develop over time, assuming baseline ability and interpersonal skills are present.

Staff value and respect clinical expertise in their manager—it adds credibility. However, clinical expertise alone will not ensure success in the role, even though it is a criterion for promotion in many organizations.

Strategies for Success

If the MNM has been promoted from within the organization, the challenge will be to supervise staff members who are friends and colleagues. The new manager has to be fair and objective and accept authority, while not appearing to abandon friendships. Yet, the new manager cannot maintain the same level of friendship with staff he or she now supervises and expect to manage effectively. The following are some strategies that are useful to the MNM.

Strategy 1: Socialize Appropriately

Be accessible and friendly, yet detached enough to be objective. Unit-based or facility functions to which all staff are invited are good ways to encourage socialization; off-site events and parties should be handled with caution for a number of reasons, including perceived favoritism, actions taken in a casual setting that you may regret, inappropriate employee interactions, and so forth.

Strategy 2: Build Your Team

Build your team by involving them in decisions, such as hiring RNs, self-scheduling, and unit-based practice improvements. Call staff meetings "team meetings." Define your expectations of teamwork and post these in the unit. Appoint small teams to unit-based projects of importance to the staff. Use the word "teamwork" frequently and praise team accomplishments.

Strategy 3: Create a Great Clinical Unit Climate

Build on what is present and acknowledge past history. Talk to each staff member about his or her perceptions and desires. Use staff meetings to set the unit-based vision and goals. Ensure that staff has the tools to get their jobs done, such as equipment, supplies, and education. Empower staff by listening, incorporating feedback, delegating, and involving them in decision making. Push all decisions to the lowest level possible and support them.

Strategy 4: Adopt a Zero Tolerance Policy for Poor Performance

Give each employee every chance to do his or her job well and contribute to the team. Counsel employees on absenteeism and tardiness. Counsel employees who have behavioral issues that affect the team. At the same time, send the message that poor performance will not be tolerated. If these measures fail, termination of employees after due process may be required. Do it!

Strategy 5: Be a Chief Retention Officer

Be proactive—know what makes your employees tick. Keep a 3 x 5 card for each that identifies what is important to him or her. Conduct an exit interview with each employee and learn from it. Track your turnover statistics. Ask staff what is important and meet their needs.

Strategy 6: Develop Yourself as a Leader

On-the-job training is not enough. Seek classes and seminars on budgetary management; performance appraisals; supervision; business plans; quality improvement; interviewing, hiring, and firing; conflict resolution; and negotiation. Ask for the tools you need, and ask for coaching from your boss. Attend local and national conferences that will enhance your managerial skills.

Strategy 7: Communicate

Communicate and communicate. Communicating with staff 24 hours a day and 7 days a week is a challenge. Try different methods such as holding staff meetings at different times and shifts; keeping team minutes in a notebook on the unit; making off-shift and weekend rounds; promoting unit newsletters; and using electronic mail, voice mail, notes on lockers, postings on bulletin boards and in the staff break room, urgent communications on brightly colored paper, "sound off" work sessions for staff, and handwritten notes. Remember: One-on-one communication is a high-touch, low-tech method that is still the most effective for communicating the needs of the unit.

Strategy 8: Give Ongoing Feedback

Recognize staff with positive feedback—praise the deed—on the work they did to make a difference. Share patient comments and letters, both positive and negative. Have staff provide feedback on colleague performance appraisals. Know your staff, and know whether they appreciate public or private praise. Provide constructive feedback when necessary and ensure that staff learn from it.

Strategy 9: Have Fun and Celebrate

Introduce fun and humor into your work area and celebrate often. Celebrate unit accomplishments with pizza parties or potluck events. Celebrate staff accomplishments with unit newsletters, postings, invitations to senior administrators to the units, small gift certificates, and parties—whatever the staff likes that can be done at work. Having physicians involved is a great way to add both fun and humor—they can cook breakfast, be an RN for a day, buy Chinese food for the staff, or provide entertainment. Hold contests, use humor in conversation, or post healthcare jokes in the staff room. Joy, fun, and celebration do make a difference in the morale of nurses.

Strategy 10: Support the Organization and Your Boss

Undermining either your boss or the organization can be career limiting. In word and deed, promote the organization and its positive attributes. Handle interpersonal SNL and MNM conflicts in private. Reject negative language such as "I can't," "I won't," and "I'll try," and replace it with positive language such as "I can," "I will," and "I have never tried that, but will give it my very best." Accept help and support from your boss and learn from each situation. Never burn bridges—you will regret it sometime in your career.

Strategy 11: Care for the Caregiver

Take care of your staff. Look for signs of burnout, such as depression, decreased interest or work performance, hopelessness, helplessness, fatigue, anger, and poor attitude. Staff need your support— it may be a one-on-one conversation, a referral to an employee assistance program, a consultation with an external facilitator on clinical units in which death and dying are commonplace, or a ten-minute break from the unit. Encourage staff to openly discuss stressful situations, provide a break area, and make sure they take the breaks that are due them. Bring in social workers or mental health professionals to teach staff deep breathing and other stress reduction techniques. Rotate difficult patient assignments between staff members. Ensure that management is present during crisis situations, especially those that are staffing related.

SUMMARY

High-performing nursing leaders create a successful organizational climate for nursing. An exceptional CNE will not achieve his or her vision without strong, cascading leadership and equally strong management. Leaders help influence all levels of staff to accomplish the goals of nursing. Nursing leaders and managers work together and complement each other. Competencies and skills required for advancement into leadership roles include emotional competencies related to emotional intelligence and concrete skills related to finance, human resource management, and strategic planning. Ineffective leadership leads to nursing turnover.

Various ways the SNL can foster a positive organizational climate were identified. Several practical and straightforward strategies for the middle manager were identified. None of the strategies or methods is difficult or magical, yet their importance is often overlooked.

Organizations need the best leaders and managers to lead the changes necessary in workforce redesign. Restructuring and redesign work is necessary to both survive and thrive in the foreseeable future and is the focus of the next chapter.

CHAPTER 11

Work Redesign: Doing the Job in a New Era

INTRODUCTION

Staffing should be based on the needs of patients. This simple concept is seldom realized because of myriad factors, including outdated productivity measures, RN shortages, inadequate methods for predicting staffing needs, decreased reimbursement, and too many demands on RN time that add little value to care of the patient.

Developing models that work in today's environment is a significant challenge. Appropriate staffing models should use available RNs effectively so that the RN feels he or she has provided quality patient care. This is a core component of retaining staff. Any model you choose must take your specific needs and the local marketplace into consideration, as well as the following questions:

- What options for nursing care delivery can be developed for your facility?
- What enablers can positively affect patient care delivery?

- When patient care redesign is necessary, how can you involve staff and make the initiative successful?

This chapter presents models that have been successful, along with strategies to involve staff. Multiple factors that affect care delivery are assessed. Results will need to be evaluated to ensure patient outcomes are not negatively affected, and patient, physician, and RN satisfaction must be monitored. These issues are also addressed.

Why redesign? Your care delivery model should be redesigned if the current one is not meeting organizational needs. For example, redesign should be considered if patient, physician, or RN satisfaction is low, the supply of RNs is inadequate, costs are too high, competitor organizations are recruiting your staff, or a new direction for nursing is being taken and redesign is an element of that process. It should be determined whether the entire organization will participate or if redesign will take place only in the nursing department.

NURSING CARE DELIVERY MODELS THAT WORK

Limited, research-based data indicate the relationship between how nursing care delivery is organized and its impact on patient outcomes and on nursing satisfaction. Scientific evidence that supports one model over another is not available. However, several factors related to this relationship must be considered when changing the care delivery model or validating the one that is being used:

- number of available RNs in your hospital; availability in your market area
- fiscal constraints; available fiscal resources to fund salaries and costs (i.e., training) associated with the model
- nursing acceptance of practice model
- expected outcomes, such as risk reduction, fewer medication errors, fewer pressure sores, improved patient satisfaction, and improved pain management

Ultimately, the goal of most patient care delivery models is to provide safe patient care at a reasonable and affordable cost. The following are commonly accepted models of nursing care delivery.

Patient-focused care: This is a model in which RNs manage a group of patients, with unlicensed assistive personnel doing task-oriented functions such as phlebotomy, electrocardiogram (EKG) tests, and basic care delivery. This works well in organizations that have the ability to fundamentally redesign patient care delivery roles. An element of chaos may occur with the implementation of this model because of complete role redesign, reapplication for positions, and changes in skill mix. Necessary components that will lead to success include planning, education, training, and ongoing evaluation.

Primary care: This model uses all staff RNs to provide care in its purest form; a modified primary care model is one variation in which other non-RN personnel are added on a limited basis. In either application of the model, the majority of care is provided by RNs. This model works well in an area in which an adequate and continuous supply of RNs is available, especially if they are baccalaureate prepared. The cost of the model is high, so the organization must be able to afford it. RNs usually are very satisfied with this care delivery model.

Team or functional: This model uses RNs as team leaders, and licensed practical or vocational nurses and aides deliver care. The work can be assigned by tasks such as patient-care treatments or medication delivery. This model works well when the supply of RNs is limited and where the setting is more traditional. RNs do tasks that only an RN can do, and others are assigned to nonlicensed personnel.

Given that no one model is proven beyond any doubt to be the best, you should select or modify the model that meets your specific needs. Many factors need to be considered in making this decision, and getting RN input and active participation in the design of your model will ensure the greatest chance of success. Factors to consider include the following:

- Job satisfaction of RNs: Do they value hands-on patient care or prefer delegation and supervision?

- Ability to recruit and retain unlicensed assistive personnel (UAP) in your environment.
- Presence or absence of nursing schools providing a continuous workforce supply.
- Ability to delegate non-patient-care activity, such as the changing of bed linens, to support departments.
- Emerging workforce (Net generation and generation X) with different employee values.
- Employment status of RN workforce—full or part time.

Developing or redesigning a care delivery model that provides personal satisfaction to RNs results in retention. Providing a model that keeps expert clinicians at the bedside is the goal.

If you are undergoing a nursing delivery model redesign, you will want to identify the rationale. Is it cost based? Is patient satisfaction low? Are your RNs dissatisfied with the current model, resulting in job dissatisfaction? Do you have an inadequate supply of RNs to make your current model work? Are adverse outcomes occuring related to care that nursing provides, such as falls, pressure sores, and medication errors?

The model that works is the one that works for you. The model must be designed for your institution. Important variables include the nursing and organizational climate, nursing and medical leadership, collaboration between physicians and nurses, availability of UAPs, support staff, RN staff, and current nursing satisfaction scores.

PROCESS STEPS FOR REDESIGN

To redesign your model, research on alternative models and staff input is critical. Ask advanced practice RNs and organizational development staff to assist. The following steps should be taken:

1. Gather data on why the redesign is necessary and ensure that all key stakeholders have a voice—use focus groups,

surveys, nursing-related patient outcomes, RN satisfaction data, etc.

2. Present the case for change in town hall meetings, staff meetings, written communications, on the intranet, and at leadership forums. Make your case in a compelling manner and seek input from staff on an ideal redesign. Use the forums to educate staff on different models and the positive and negative aspects of each.

3. Design the characteristics of the new system. Use all levels of nursing personnel in the design process—RNs, advanced practice nurses, UAPs, and managers. Often, a draft redesign can be used to seek input and can then be refined and revised. Incorporate characteristics of the ideal design. Commit the characteristics to paper after input from a broad nursing audience.

4. Take preliminary design characteristics to your staff for feedback. Poster boards can be displayed throughout the hospital facility. As dialog continues, the new model should become clear.

5. Design the new model and present it to staff for final input before the implementation rolls out. Make final revisions, estimate the cost of the model, and seek CEO endorsement.

6. Develop an implementation plan, with key tasks, time lines, and accountabilities assigned. Use planning software. Prepare milestone checks throughout the project to ensure it is on track.

As your redesign task force looks at ways to enhance the delivery model, present ideas to them to determine which works best for you.

Do You Want a Model that Reassigns Nonclinical Tasks?

If a model that reassigns nonclinical tasks is the goal, determine whether these tasks need to be assigned to support departments, if support department personnel need to be assigned to nursing, or if new types of assistive workers should be recruited.

Do You Want a Model that Uses Nonprofessional Support Staff for the Delegation of Tasks?

If a model that delegates to nonprofessional support staff is the goal, evaluate the feasibility of pairing an RN with a nonlicensed care partner to assist with the nurse's work. The care partnership may replace two RNs with one RN and one UAP, assuming care for a caseload of patients is covered.

An alternative is to have several RNs supervise a group of non-partnered UAPs. This group is assigned tasks and helps with task completion.

How to Involve Staff in Redesign

Restructuring and reengineering were the prevalent cost management trends in the 1990s and still continue to be used. Hospitals and health systems are facing reimbursement declines at the same time that wages are escalating because of marketplace shortages. Any redesign or restructuring requires leaders who can be change agents and staff who can adapt to change.

First and foremost, nursing leaders need to embrace the change and be able to effectively handle it. Goleman (1998) identifies the change catalyst in the social skills competency within emotional intelligence. Leaders with this competence can not only survive restructuring or redesign, but have a department that excels and exceeds expectations.

Leaders with this competence:

1. see the need for the change and remove the barriers,
2. challenge the status quo and identify the need for the change,

3. serve as champions of the change and inspire others, and

4. serve as a role model by exhibiting the expected behaviors.

Inform staff of the vision and rationale for the redesign to get them involved and enthusiastic about it. This involves your abilities to influence, listen to resistance, manage through the politics, persevere, and show enthusiasm.

Be a homeowner, not a renter. The workplace is your home away from home, so make a commitment. Owners are committed; renters are passing through.

Key Success Factors

A number of key success factors will enable the redesign process to succeed. None are difficult, and most are needed. Do not be afraid to change or modify the design while in implementation. You may not know what revisions are required until you test the design.

1. Make the case for change in nursing forums, in letters to staff, to nursing leadership, and in nursing newsletters. Use "talking points" for your leadership group so the message can be consistent: create a summary of the key points in bulleted form so that everyone speaks to the same key points.

2. Appoint a design team composed of staff, managers, advance practice RNs, and educators. Designate an experienced team leader and a team facilitator. Give them the parameters of the desired outcomes, such as improved patient satisfaction, reduced cost, increased overall care hours, reduced RN skill mix, or improved nursing satisfaction.

3. Provide resources for the team, such as an external consultant, articles, summaries of various patient care delivery systems, staff from other facilities who have been successful, and site visits.

4. Identify the measurement plan. Factors to be measured may include decrease in worked nursing hours per patient day, decrease in RN skill mix, increase in patient satisfaction, or decrease in cost per patient day.
5. After completing the preliminary design, test it on staff focus groups for input. Revise as needed.
6. Communicate, communicate, communicate. Keep all staff apprised of progress throughout the process and continue to give and accept feedback.
7. Test the design on a single nursing unit. Criteria for selection include a stable RN staff, an enthusiastic manager (preferably from the design team), a supportive physician leader and collaborative physician-nurse relationships, history of adaptability and flexibility, and willingness to be first.
8. Implement the redesign organizationwide, using design team members and staff from the pilot units to describe their experiences, educate staff, motivate staff, and assuage staff fears.
9. Monitor results; hold managers accountable for the success of the redesign.
10. Evaluate overall results and clinical unit results.
11. Support and coach departments with mixed results until success is assured.
12. Evaluate the redesign once per quarter during year one of implementation to ensure change is maintained.

RN work redesign can be more focused and based on identified issues that dissatisfy staff. Projects can be tackled at the unit or sectional level or for the organization.

Redesign results important to the nursing staff that should be considered in the new model include the following:

- more time for direct patient care
- reduction of paperwork
- timely medication delivery from the pharmacy

- support staff responsiveness to patient needs from such areas as housekeeping, maintenance, and food service
- reduction of nonnursing tasks such as delivering food trays, changing linens, stocking supplies, and procuring results from multiple departments
- improved communication systems, such as wireless phones, walkie-talkies, text messaging, etc.
- medication and support procurement and charging systems (the system of charging items used in patient care to the patient)

Implementing a project on the unit level can be very beneficial to staff morale. By having staff form a small team within the clinical unit to tackle and resolve issues, time spent on patient care can be increased if they are successful at identifying improvements. Other departments can be added if the issue is multidisciplinary.

Aside from an overall redesign of patient care delivery, staff should be involved in the redesign of their own unit-based work relating to patient care delivery. For example, a clinical excellence council could be formed that would focus on improving clinical practice, developing protocols for target patient populations, and improving resident physician and nurse collaborative practice. Staff will be able to identify and embrace their ability to positively affect patient care.

SKILL MIX ISSUES

We know that better staffing leads to better outcomes, but we cannot always afford additional staffing or even find the staff. Given these conflicting data, a fundamental decision must be made at the beginning of the redesign process about your philosophy on the skill mix and the type of model selected. Even if you choose a high RN skill mix akin to the primary care model, which in its purest form is an all-RN caregiving model, you may want a small percentage of workers to support the primary RN. If you want a balanced skill mix, decide which model will work best in terms of how unlicensed staff are used.

A working paper by Gillow (2002) identifies issues for consideration when using unlicensed caregiver staff:

- RNs who do not supervise unlicensed caregiver staff may be up to 25 percent more productive.
- Fifty percent of unlicensed caregiver staff may be unproductive as they are waiting to be told what to do and then what to do next.

Figure 11.1: *(continued)*

Process/Steps
- Steering group composed of managers and staff selected
- Work teams given assignments, timelines, and available resources. Teams related to documentation, standards of care and practice, development of mission and vision, design of nursing report card, and patient care delivery model
- Literature review, Internet searches, and telephone interviews completed from targeted hospitals with successful redesign
- Design of nursing report card
- Design of implementation plan, communication, and roll out

Components
- Nursing mission and vision
- Standards of care and standards of professional practice
- Point-of-care documentation
- Patient care delivery model composed of RNs and unlicensed assistive personnel
- Redesign of nursing management and support roles
- Design of nursing report card

Source: Advocate Lutheran General Hospital, Chicago, IL. Used with permission.

- Almost 25 percent of an RN's time is spent providing instruction to unlicensed staff, following up, and assessing delegated work thus taking time away from direct RN patient care.

For models using unlicensed staff to be effective, education for your RN staff is needed on delegation and streamlined processes and protocols, including streamlined documentation. Unlicensed workers who have little opportunity for upward mobility without additional education need support, need to feel valued, and should also have horizontal career mobility. As their skills expand, consider level I and level II UAP roles so they have promotional opportunities. Figure 11.1 is a template of an overall nursing redesign model used at Advocate Lutheran General Hospital, a large, tertiary medical center in the Chicago metropolitan area.

BUILDING AN ALIGNED NURSING STAFF

While the type of care delivery model is important to identify, other factors should also be considered. Mission, vision, and values have been discussed earlier in the book. Recall that nursing needs a vision to describe what nursing is related to its scope of practice, provision of care, governance, organization of competency assessment, staffing and scheduling, quality improvement and quality assurance, documentation systems, and growth and development.

A common vision, set of values, and set of goals create staff alignment. Alignment of the nursing staff with a professional practice model can be developed in a single hospital or across hospitals. It is best to start from scratch and not attempt modest change that has little impact. Fundamental redesign around components of professional nursing practice can motivate and inspire staff by ensuring their involvement in the issues affecting their nursing practice.

USING INFORMATION TECHNOLOGY

Technology in the healthcare industry used for patient care delivery and the practice of nursing lags behind other industries. Given that generation X and Net generation staff expect to use technology, the technologically advanced organization has a competitive edge in recruitment and retention. Healthcare and nursing organizations collect a great deal of data, yet information is often not available to nursing staff. Data needs are seldom analyzed to determine if they actually add value or are required for regulatory bodies. A good exercise is to review all data collected within the nursing arena and for what purpose. Then analyze the criticality of the data and determine if data collection and reporting must continue, can be discontinued, or can be streamlined. Time spent on data collection can be reduced by doing this simple exercise.

Automation of data may help, if those data have a purpose and the automation facilitates nursing work, improves patient care, provides trending data that can be used to improve practice, or is useful in managing the nursing enterprise. Be aware that even when data are automated, the new system may not be used to its potential and may increase work because of data entry requirements.

Nurses spend an average of 30 minutes or more on the regulatory burden of paperwork for the average Medicare patient. More than 100 regulations affecting healthcare have passed since 1997 (Paolucci 2001). Much of the data are not used in a meaningful way to affect patient outcomes.

Clinical information systems are the focus of a great deal of attention and are recommended in the Institute of Medicine (1999) report as a way of increasing patient safety. They also have gained attention in the media because some insurers are beginning to require a commitment on the part of healthcare providers to implement these systems in order to be on the preferred provider list and continue to be in the insurer's network.

Without carefully evaluating, planning, and implementing these systems and understanding the true return on investment, you may be disappointed in the ability of information technology to meet your expectations. However, clinical information systems can assist the RN in being more efficient and effective, especially if all systems are networked and many manual processes disappear. One of the most effective ways to streamline RN time and reduce risk to patients is with physician order entry and an integrated network of clinical systems that "talk" to each other. Having immediate access to clinical information from a variety of sources helps the RN do his or her job and better assist the physician in optimal patient care delivery.

Although information technology does not solve all of nursing's issues, it can provide invaluable assistance to the RN practice, to effective patient care delivery, to administrative management, and to education. Increasingly, hospitals are turning to technology to improve the way work is done.

Technology that Supports Nursing Practice

Systems that are often most beneficial to RNs include the following:

1. Automated medication dispensing systems that distribute, track, and bill medications and interface with pharmacy
2. Automated supply towers at the unit level that dispense, track, and bill and are tied into materials management
3. Clinical documentation systems that enable RNs to chart efficiently and retrieve data for trending and improving patient care
4. Patient care monitoring systems and devices such as infusion pumps and ventilators that interface with documentation systems
5. Physician order entry systems that markedly reduce the paperwork and rework inherent in carrying out orders and that reduce medication errors and delays in treatment
6. Wireless technology communication systems such as wireless telephones and pagers that enable better communication and messaging
7. Sophisticated patient call systems that have call-in stations and patient-to-RN interaction features
8. Locator systems with "search and find" features that reduce RN time in locating other staff, equipment, and off-unit patients

Technology that Supports Nursing Education

Classroom education still has a role, but increasingly RNs are being taught in an interactive and self-directed way using technology via the Internet, distance learning, and CD-ROM. Nurses can learn at home, on the unit when there is down time, on a personal computer that can be anywhere, or in a nursing education center equipped with computers and the latest technology.

Nurses can react to clinical situations and ethical issues, learn new policies and procedures, complete required testing and education, take courses on myriad clinical topics ranging from cardiac arrhythmias to advanced oncology, and complete certification courses. The new way of teaching is more cost effective, allows learners to pace themselves, and provides ongoing support and feedback. It is a way of life for the Net generation and generation X employees and is usually easy for the baby boomers in your workplace to learn. Be sure to have an educator or support RN present for staff who are not computer literate and fearful of using the technology.

Technology that Supports Nursing Management

Automation is very helpful to the business of nursing. A personal computer is a basic tool that each middle nurse manager (MNM) should have available. Automation can assist in staffing and scheduling, RN license tracking, mandatory education, competency tracking, cardiopulmonary resuscitation (CPR) training tracking, and tracking of dates you wish to remember. If you do not know how to use a computer, take a course at a local community college, through your information systems department, at your local library, or through an outside vendor.

Performance appraisals can be automated, or at least typed and saved in a software program on the computer. Optimally, the performance appraisal can be completed online; when submitted and approved, the accompanying pay rate adjustment can occur automatically. Performance feedback is important to employees, and automation assists you with getting it done on time.

Another automated system that is very beneficial is one that helps you manage time and attendance. This enables tracking of RN hours and ensures appropriate pay. It tracks absences, time off for illness, and holiday or vacation time off and allows trending over time. It can help identify issues with overtime or bonus pay and quickly flags irregular pay practices.

Automation may be homegrown, using simple spreadsheets, databases, or software, or may be purchased from specialized outside vendors. These do no have to be complicated. Almost every MNM can develop them on his or her own after a basic personal computer course or two. Community colleges, libraries, and businesses offer inexpensive one-day courses on basic computer skills, spreadsheets, and other applications.

Information technology enablers are increasingly critical to efficient and effective patient care delivery and management because they enable nurses to reduce the time spent on paperwork, phone calls to track missing medications, phone calls to physicians for orders, and related non-direct-care activities. Some technology enablers include physician order enty, medication dispensing systems, and wireless communication systems. Manual processes create risk to patients, especially related to medication administration. Too many opportunities for errors are present, and medication near misses and sentinel events are problems in even the best hospitals in the country.

Manual processes also create opportunities for error in the way RNs are managed. This can lead to dissatisfaction among your staff. RNs deserve to be paid correctly, scheduled in a way that is fair and consistent, and assured that they have the education and competency to do the job.

SUMMARY

This chapter focuses on work redesign and strategies and steps that will help ensure success in that process. Involving staff every step of the way and aligning staff around components of professional practice are essential to the buy-in of redesign and are part of an effective strategy for recruiting and retaining nurses.

Work redesign should be an ongoing initiative to meet the needs of patient care delivery and to continually improve processes related to nursing care. Technology is an enabler that can positively affect nursing practice and management. Automating clinical and administrative processes can improve productivity, streamline managerial processes, and enable improvements in patient care. Technology is a critical success factor and should be optimally used within the nursing arena.

This section concludes with Appendix 11.1, "Toolbox: 100 Ways to Lead."

REFERENCES

Gillow, K. 2002. "Organizing the Nursing Work Force: A Review of the Literature." Working paper. [Online publication; retrieved Feb. 20, 2002.] Washington, DC: American Nurses Association. www.fhs.mcmaster.ca/nru/old%20nru/html /papers.html.

Goleman, D. 1998. *Working with Emotional Intelligence*, Appendix 1, pp. 317–18. New York: Bantam Books.

Institute of Medicine. 1999. *To Err is Human: Building a Safer Health System*, edited by L. T. Kohn, J. M. Corrigan, and M. S. Donaldson. Washington, DC: National Academy Press.

Paolucci, M. 2001. "More RNs on Staff to Lower Hospital Costs." *NurseWeek*. [Online article; retrieved Sept. 27, 2002.] Washington, DC: American Nurses Association. www.nurseweek.com/nursingshortage/5-07news.html.

APPENDIX 11.1
TOOLBOX: 100 WAYS TO LEAD

Communicating

1. Visit employees on all shifts.
2. Hold town hall meetings at least quarterly.
3. Publish a monthly newsletter for all staff related to hospital and nursing news, continuing education, job openings, and celebrations.
4. Hold breakfast or lunch meetings with new employees that are informal, designed to "break the ice," and provide open dialog.
5. Complete quarterly or biannual nursing associate satisfaction surveys; provide feedback to all staff by clinical unit.
6. Repeat your message over and over, and use many different vehicles.
7. Develop a mechanism for employees to express their concerns; ask them questions requiring a direct response, or ask them through the human resources department to protect their confidentiality, if they do not want their name used.
8. Use humor and storytelling to make your points.
9. Learn when to "zip your lip"—sometimes it is better to sit on a critical comment or email for at least 24 hours.
10. Never use capital letters in electronic mail—it is a form of electronic yelling.
11. Use electronic mail for getting out urgent messages quickly—circumvent the grapevine.
12. Use the in-house television channel to educate employees around the clock.
13. Send a letter to each employee's home to notify him or her of breaking news, positive or negative, in language that is easy to understand.
14. Show trust in your staff by sharing financial information and other key indicators.

15. Show that you value and embrace work-life-family balance in word and deed.
16. Have RN staff write letters of welcome to new employees.
17. Use scripts for customer satisfaction or key employee communications.
18. Use quotes from famous leaders—find these on the Internet, at book stores, and at libraries.
19. Use gestures, body language, and speech to get your point across.
20. Never react or over-react to criticism, anger, resistance, or sarcastic responses—listen and reflect; empathize with the employee.

Leading

21. Assign managers and directors to areas other than their own for making rounds and to increase management visibility.
22. Be on site and visible in times of crisis: layoffs, restructuring, high census, and sentinel events.
23. Lead by example—be a positive and enthusiastic role model.
24. Admit when you are wrong and apologize.
25. Frequently ask, "how can I help you?" or "what do you need from me?"
26. Seek frequent feedback on your performance from your boss, direct reports, colleagues, physicians, and staff.
27. Demonstrate your commitment to staff by coaching, mentoring, providing learning opportunities, and setting "stretch goals" for your staff.
28. Wander around, bring good news, talk on a personal level.
29. Be where you are least expected—a quality meeting, a very busy weekend shift, a unit celebration, etc.
30. Hold all of your staff accountable consistently.
31. Start every management meeting with a celebration moment.

32. Assign each new manager or director a mentor; provide experienced managers and directors with a mentor in a different area if it promotes career growth and development.
33. Always have a succession plan for all management levels.
34. Actively seek out staff with leadership potential and groom them for the next step in their career path.
35. Provide sabbaticals to your most talented staff, with a focus on returning to the organization with new skill, competency, or knowledge.
36. Provide renewal opportunities for your management team via retreats, changes to the portfolios they manage, mentoring opportunities, and leadership courses.
37. Send the message that poor performance will not be tolerated—terminate poor performers after a development plan for improvement has failed.
38. Find common ground in a conflict situation and build on it.
39. Never ask others to do what you are unwilling to do yourself.
40. Never accept the status quo—always challenge and always look for ways to improve. Ask your staff—they will tell you where to look.

Showcasing

41. Publicly recognize your staff—be sure they get credit for their achievements.
42. Promote from within or provide new assignments outside of the current management area.
43. Hold contests—let managers and staff compete for prizes and showcase the winners. Hold a theme-based nursing poster contest, a holiday decorating contest, a "name that physician" contest using baby pictures, a contest for a theme for Nurses' Week. Be creative.

44. Send handwritten notes to staff and managers who go above and beyond and recognize them in meetings.
45. Hold a team recognition function such as an ice cream or pizza party for the best patient satisfaction, the best nursing satisfaction, or other achievements.
46. Use storytelling publicity to recognize your heroes and heroines.
47. Showcase personnel or a clinical department by taking external visitors to the area, notifying the media, or having them make a presentation in front of a hospital forum.
48. Look for young stars—talk to them one on one and solicit their ideas; increase their visibility by special clinical unit assignments.
49. Look at every person you hire as a possible successor—hire the brightest and the best.
50. Give a trophy or a banner to high-performing nursing units or departments.

Changing

51. Share the vision, share the plan.
52. Involve employees and let them provide feedback and help in the planning.
53. Allow time for grieving and resistance—be visible, let people vent, and explain it over and over.
54. Communicate your plan to the target audience and all other constituencies that will be affected (i.e., physicians, other departments, external community groups, etc.).
55. Be willing to give each staff member the opportunity and tools to change, but do not allow resistors to stay after coaching and training fail.

56. Hire staff who embrace change—look for these characteristics in the interview process or on the resume.
57. Be consistent—do not allow a return to the old method. Have a ceremony to bury the old, or take away all opportunities for slippage.
58. Clearly show over and over what the change is and how it will benefit the staff.
59. Speak with a consistent voice—cascade a major change throughout the organization by using talking points and scripts.
60. Pilot a new idea before you implement on a full scale—redesign as needed.

Teambuilding

61. Delegate, and then get out of the way.
62. Eliminate "me" from your vocabulary, substitute it with "we."
63. Hire team players—let the team do the interviewing and selection.
64. Hold team-building management and staff retreats, even if you only have two hours available.
65. Create teams for special assignments: clinical excellence, patient satisfaction, cost management, associate satisfaction, or work redesign.
66. Celebrate team victories.
67. Offer many company-sponsored team opportunities and events: bowling, sports teams, talent show and theater.
68. Hold silly and fun events for your staff—have fun at the clinical unit level or facilitywide.
69. Measure and reward team performance on an ongoing basis.
70. Give small rewards, such as video gift certificates, fast food or coffee shop coupons, book store coupons, or cash, to team members at milestones in a project.

71. Provide assessment and intervention to dysfunctional teams. Human resources, education, or organizational development areas can assist in getting the team on track.
72. Assess each team meeting. Ask each participant to identify "did well" and "could improve."
73. Give frequent feedback to your teams.
74. Charter highly focused, short-term teams to do a specific function. When completed, disband the group and reward members.
75. Let teams design their workspace—break rooms, conference rooms, and unit work areas.
76. When a manager resigns, work with employees and empower them to function as a self-directed work team.
77. Introduce self-scheduling to a high-performing nursing unit—identify guidelines and let nurses schedule hours to meet personal needs, while taking into consideration patient care needs.
78. Provide stress management sessions for teams in distress. Internal resources such as chaplains, social workers, or psychologists can help teams cope with specific stressors or provide stress management techniques.
79. Know the signs of a well-functioning team: high participation, decisions by consensus, results-oriented participants, and positive energy.

Developing/Growing

80. Attend national and local professional organization meetings.
81. Get involved in local groups of healthcare or specialty managers.
82. Read healthcare and nursing management literature.
83. Attend one unique seminar annually that will enhance your critical thinking abilities or skills.

84. Scan the healthcare- and nursing-related web sites.
85. Network with professional colleagues.
86. Read at least one new leadership concept book and listen to one management audiotape every quarter.
87. Obtain newsletters via the Internet or mail related to your clinical specialty or management area.
88. Ask for special assignments outside of your usual area of expertise.
89. Step into the void—volunteer to do a difficult task and produce results.
90. Ask for 360-degree feedback on your performance.
91. Hire a personal career coach if you are struggling professionally.
92. Be self-directed—do not ask, just do, when you see something that needs to be done.
93. Assess your growth needs and develop a plan, be it on public speaking, business plans, fiscal management, etc.
94. Take a college- or graduate-level course to enhance your education and learning.
95. Pursue a degree in a field of interest to you.
96. Write an article for publication, even if you have never done so.
97. Volunteer in your professional organization, in the workplace, and in the community—build your network and increase your visibility.
98. Learn from your mistakes—analyze what you did wrong and how to improve the next time.
99. Create a career path for yourself.
100. Identify a mentor and develop a long-term relationship. Look outside of nursing, as well as within the field.

PART V

Nursing Rx for the Present and Future

CHAPTER 12

Magnet Status and Its Impact on Nurse Recruitment and Retention

INTRODUCTION

One of the positive trends in nursing has been the creation of the Magnet Nursing Services Recognition Program for Excellence in Nursing Services. The program is the highest level of recognition that the American Nurses Credentialing Center can provide to organized nursing services in healthcare organizations (*Nursing World* 2002b).

The Magnet Nursing Services Recognition Program for Excellence in Nursing Services grew out of a 1982 descriptive study conducted by the American Academy of Nursing's Task Force on Nursing Practice (*Nursing World* 2002b). The study, conducted in 41 hospitals, identified and described variables that created an environment that attracted and retained well-qualified nurses who provided excellence in nursing services and thus promoted quality patient care. These institutions were termed "magnet" hospitals because they attracted and retained professional nurses who experienced professional and personal satisfaction in their practice (McClure et al. 1983).

The researchers began by identifying a national sample of magnet hospitals. Nursing fellows from the American Academy of Nursing were asked to nominate potential magnet hospitals from their region. Their nominations were based on three criteria:

1. The nurses considered the hospital a good place to practice nursing and work.
2. The hospital had a low turnover rate.
3. The hospital competed for nursing staff with other institutions and agencies.

The fellows nominated a total of 165 institutions. The task force then began narrowing the list based on specific criteria and the hospitals' willingness and availability to participate. After identifying the 41 hospitals, the researchers held group interviews. One session was held with directors of nursing and another with staff nurses. Nurses were asked nine questions, which remain valuable for structuring nurse input even today:

1. What makes your hospital a good place for nurses to work?
2. Can you describe particular programs that you see leading to professional/personal satisfaction?
3. How is nursing viewed in your hospital, and why?
4. Can you describe nurse involvement in various ongoing programs/projects whose goals are quality of patient care?
5. Can you identify activities and programs calculated to enhance, both directly and indirectly, recruitment/retention of professional nurses in your hospital?
6. Could you tell us about nurse-physician relationships in your hospital?
7. Describe staff nurse–supervisor relationships in your hospital.
8. Are some areas in your hospital more successful than others in recruitment/retention? Why?
9. What single piece of advice would you give to a director of nursing who wishes to do something about high RN vacancy and turnover rates in his or her hospital?

The findings are telling. Staff nurses identified a variety of conditions that made a hospital a good place for nurses to work that were categorized into administration, professional practice, and professional development. Information was reported as the staff nurses' conceptions of the conditions that make a hospital a good place for nurses to work. All generalizations were derived from the staff nurses' comments (McClure et al. 1983). The discussion that follows is based on the findings of McClure et al. (1983).

ADMINISTRATION

During their interviews, staff nurses in magnet hospitals indicated that a positive work environment was related to nursing administration. They specifically mentioned management style, quality of leadership, organizational structure, staffing, and personnel policies and programs.

Management Style

Staff nurses indicated clearly that the nursing leaders were important to a hospital's magnetism. The magnet hospital nurses described visible and accessible nursing leaders and the use of participatory management.

Visibility and Accessibility

Nurse executives were visible in the institutions and accessible for support and problem resolution. They made rounds on patient units, talked to staff nurses, discussed patient and nursing problems, listened to staff nurses, and responded to what nurses said. They set the tone for nursing at the institution: they participated in orientation, described the philosophy of nursing, and recognized the staff nurses for their accomplishments. Nurse executives recognized the autonomy of the staff nurses and provided support through resources such as clinical nurse specialists, managers, and supervisors. Nurse executives also encouraged nurses in self-development.

Participatory Management

Management was viewed as participatory, with staff nurses actively engaged in decision making at the unit, department, and hospital levels. Staff nurses reported being involved in many aspects of the organization, including evaluating and selecting new equipment and patient care supply items, planning for new services, designing new patient care areas, developing computerized patient information systems, planning quality programs, and creating health education programs for patients and community members. Communications were open between management and staff and used a variety of channels, including individual interactions, group meetings, committees, newsletters, and surveys.

Quality of Leadership

Magnet hospital staff nurses indicated that nursing leaders served as top executives in the hospital and represented the needs of nursing in an articulate manner. They described the strength and knowledge of nursing leaders, administrative support, and administrative expectations.

Strength and Knowledge

Staff nurses viewed a key role of nurse executives as the articulation of a clear philosophy based on the importance of caring for patients, family, and self. Nurse executives were viewed as strong nurse advocates, expecting staff nurses to deliver high-quality care at controlled costs. Staff nurses were educated about budget issues and expected nurse executives to prevent crippling cuts in the nursing budget and to ensure the required nursing staff and programs for quality care. Staff nurses were also encouraged to work effectively with people from other departments.

Administrative Support

Nurse executives were perceived as providing care and support to staff nurses. They put tactics in place to relieve nurse burden and improve work life quality, such as satellite pharmacies, night cafeteria hours, and psychological consultation for staff. In addition, the nurse executive supported the staff nurse in his or her role as patient advocate when questionable medical care was identified.

Staff nurses praised the support and leadership they received from effective and knowledgeable nurse managers and supervisors. Supervisors were described as valuable, visible, and accessible and were viewed as an important safety net in emergencies. Nurse managers were perceived as extremely important in achieving and maintaining nurse satisfaction. The managers promoted, facilitated, and supported autonomy and accountability for the nursing staff. From the staff nurse perspective, the nurse managers' effectiveness played a key role in retention of staff. Other variables that were described as affecting retention included interpersonal relationships on the unit, concern for individual staff needs and interests, degree of staff involvement in unit affairs, problem solving, and quality patient care. The nurse manager was perceived as instrumental in the continuing development of staff nurses. A clean and well-maintained physical plant also contributed to the hospital's appeal as a good place to work.

Administrative Expectations

The total atmosphere in these magnet hospitals was perceived as positive. High standards were clearly articulated and administrative support was provided to ensure that the standards were met. Nurse executives expected nurses to grow and seek additional information. For example, financial support was provided for continued formal education.

Organizational Structure

An organizational structure contributes to the ambience of the hospital and provides the framework in which nurses practice. In magnet hospitals, a good relationship existed between administration and staff, with a focus on collaboration to achieve the hospital's mission. Responsibilities were decentralized to the patient care units. Organizational matters, such as scheduling, assignments, and educational activities, were handled collaboratively by the nurse manager and the staff. Committees played a key role in energizing the nursing staff in hospital and nursing issues. In particular, joint practice committees, with nurses and physicians, were viewed positively and were felt to enhance nurse satisfaction as well as quality of care.

Staffing

The magnet hospitals had a low patient-to-RN ratio, with adequate staff to provide nursing care to all patients. The quality and complexity of patient care needs were considered in staffing decisions. Staff nurses expressed great satisfaction in their ability to provide good care and in administration's support for it; they did not feel overworked and had the opportunity to address psychological and interpersonal needs as well as physical needs. Staff nurses also appreciated the availability of nurse specialists for consultation and the high RN-to-nonprofessional ratio. Float pools were identified as important in maintaining adequate staffing with registered nurses. As float pools are specific to the hospital, they ensure a consistent level of care and preclude the use of outside agency nurses.

Personnel Policies and Programs

Staff nurses in magnet hospitals were very positive about personnel policies and programs. They viewed themselves as involved in decisions and identified a variety of approaches used to meet both hospitals' and nurses' needs. The nurses described work schedules, salaries and benefits, recruitment and retention, and social recognition programs.

Schedules

Flexible schedules to accommodate individual needs were very important to the magnet hospital nurses. The nurses expressed a need to minimize the conflict between the professional and personal areas of their life. Nurses appreciated the opportunity to work with their nurse manager to plan their work schedules, with consideration given to arranging hours to accommodate family needs, educational programs, and other personal preferences. Such flexibility was accomplished with the use of 8-, 10-, and 12-hour shifts and the hiring of full-time, part-time, and float pool staff. Weekends were important for most nurses. A variety of strategies were in place to minimize the number of weekends each nurse needed to work, including weekend differentials and weekend staff who worked 24 hours and were paid for 40 hours. Shift rotation was also minimized through incentive programs.

Salaries and Benefits

Most magnet hospital nurses indicated that their salaries were competitive with those of other hospitals in their area. Some nurses indicated their hospitals provided salary bonuses for retention, night duty, increased education, clinical expertise, and overtime. Magnet hospital nurses also described benefits positively, including health insurance, dental and eye care, tuition reimbursement, child care, and three to four weeks of vacation. Some institutions had initiated cafeteria-style benefits, allowing nurses to select the benefits that best met their needs. The pooling of vacation, holiday time, and sick time into one paid-time-off pool was also viewed positively by staff nurses.

Recruitment and Retention

Magnet hospital staff nurses viewed themselves as playing a role in their hospital's organized programs for recruitment. They indicated that staff nurses were the best recruiters, serving as tour guides and small group discussion leaders at open houses. Many preferred that nurse recruiters themselves be registered nurses. Nurse recruitment committees were in place in some hospitals; staff nurses were involved in visiting nursing schools, participating in health fairs, and staffing booths at conventions.

A variety of recruitment incentives were mentioned, including scholarships or interest-free loans to nursing students in return for a committed period of employment, bonuses to employees who recruit a staff nurse, and payment for relocation expenses. Nurse extern programs were also described as a recruitment tool. In these programs, students who had completed their junior year in a bachelor of nursing program were employed during the summer months and on weekends during the school year. The programs provided a rich recruitment source.

Hospital reputation was identified as important for successful recruitment. Magnet hospitals typically had excellent reputations for both medical and nursing care, drawing nurses to them. Unique features of the hospitals were also perceived as enhancing recruitment. Shock/trauma units, high-risk obstetric treatment, rural hospitals, and university hospitals were mentioned as unique features that drew in nurses.

Social Recognition Programs

Recognition programs for outstanding contributions were common and often involved a social activity like a luncheon. Wide visibility and recognition were provided to the individuals involved. Staff nurses also mentioned social events that facilitated interactions with other nurses and other department employees as contributing to a positive environment in their hospitals. Activities included sports teams, dinners, dances, exercise programs, and self-improvement classes.

PROFESSIONAL PRACTICE

Opportunities for professional practice and the quality of that practice were perceived by the nurses as two of the most important factors contributing to the magnetism of the hospitals. The staff nurses described quality of care, professional models of care, autonomy, quality assurance, consultation and resources, community and the hospital, nurses as teachers, the image of nursing, and nurse-physician relationships.

Quality of Care

Throughout the interviews, staff nurses focused on concern for nursing practice and the factors that affect the delivery of quality care. Nurses indicated they needed the opportunity to provide high-quality care and emphasized the satisfaction derived from being able to practice nursing.

Professional Models of Care

Primary care nursing was the preferred model, and nurses used terms such as holistic care, family-centered care, and a professional model of care. In general, the nurses wanted and accepted the concept of 24-hour accountability for their patients in a setting where they could meet the total needs of their patients and evaluate the results of their practice. Primary care nursing was viewed as facilitating interdisciplinary planning and coordination of care. Staff nurses described discharge planning conferences and patient-family health education programs as examples of the collaboration and autonomy possible in this model.

Autonomy

Nurses viewed nursing care of patients as the core function of the hospital. They indicated that primary care nursing allowed independent judgment and freedom to function. The nurse was viewed as the center of communication and information. Nurses viewed themselves as particularly autonomous in settings with no or few resident physicians.

Quality Assurance

At the time of the research by McClure and colleagues, continuous quality improvement and quality management programs had not moved from other industries into healthcare. Quality assurance programs were viewed as very constructive. Staff nurses expressed the belief that involvement of nursing staff in quality assurance programs would result in improved nursing care. The nurses valued the accountability associated with the review and evaluation of nursing care. Nursing audits generated a feeling of pride.

Consultation and Resources

Staff nurses recognized the need for and appropriately used a support system. They identified the nurse manager, supervisor, and clinical nurse specialist as key support and resource people. Additional resources cited included psychiatric liaison nurses, an ethicist, and representatives of other healthcare disciplines. Colleagues were also used for consultation.

Community and the Hospital

Many of the magnet hospital staff nurses viewed professional practice as extending out to the community. They were aware of the extension of inpatient care into the community and of existing programs to promote health in the community. Nurses were very proud of their role in helping to improve the health of the community, particularly when they themselves had developed a community program.

Nurses as Teachers

Magnet hospital staff nurses indicated that they derived satisfaction from teaching. They wanted to make a contribution to teaching patients and families, viewed teaching nurses and other healthcare providers as a professional obligation, and considered teaching an aspect of their own professional growth and advancement. Thus, they reported teaching nursing students, nurses, medical students, interns, residents, patients, families, and community members. They enjoyed serving as preceptors and role models. They used a variety of media, including videotaping, audiotaping, and distribution of pamphlet materials. They taught in groups and individually. They valued their role as teacher.

The Image of Nursing

Nurses were alert to the image of nursing in their hospitals. Nurses were recognized as being knowledgeable and for the quality of their nursing care. They felt respected by patients, families, the community, physicians, other departments, and other nurses.

Nurse-Physician Relationships

Magnet hospital staff nurses indicated that a positive nurse-physician relationship was important for professional satisfaction. Although they acknowledged room for improvement, in general the relationship was described as good or excellent. They perceived mutual respect for each other's knowledge and competence and a mutual concern for the provision of quality patient care.

PROFESSIONAL DEVELOPMENT

Staff nurses valued continuing professional development and viewed it as essential to quality care and career advancement. They considered this professional development to be a responsibility of administration and a major element in their personnel benefits package. They described many opportunities for professional growth, including orientation, in-service programs, continuing and formal education, and career development.

Orientation

All magnet hospital staff nurses reported good orientation programs. The programs lasted a few weeks to several months and included formal class work, orientation to the hospital's policies, and an extended period of clinical practice, often with a preceptor. Orientations were viewed as valuable for both the new nurse and the experienced transfer nurse. The nurses were enthusiastic about preceptor programs and mentioned the training they received to assume the role.

In-service Education

Staff nurses indicated that in-service education was available to meet personal needs, interests, and objectives. In addition to traditional didactic lectures, self-directed programs and learning modules were available. Nurses identified their own learning needs and sought appropriate education. Often, staff nurses indicated that the hospitals provided in-service education as part of their career ladder.

Continuing Education

Continuing education was viewed as another mechanism for personal and professional growth. Continuing education, both on and off site, was supported by the hospitals. Some institutions required a certain number of continuing education units each year.

Formal Education

Staff nurses were enthusiastic about their hospital's attitudes toward higher education. They felt encouraged to pursue a baccalaureate degree, with on-site counseling available in some cases. Magnet hospitals made some accommodations in scheduling and provided leaves to assist staff nurses in completing their degrees. Tuition reimbursement and some scholarships were also available.

Career Development

Magnet hospital staff nurses perceived career ladders as being an essential part of professional development. They perceived ladders as a personal benefit and an educational program for professional growth and career development. Most magnet hospitals already had career ladders in place or were planning them. Nurses cited career ladders as allowing nurses to advance in recognition and salary while still continuing in clinical practice. Several nurses also mentioned a management/administration career ladder, enabling staff nurses to move into the roles of nurse manager and supervisor.

THE MAGNET NURSING SERVICES RECOGNITION PROGRAM FOR EXCELLENCE IN NURSING SERVICES

After the original magnet study results were published by McClure and colleagues in 1983, the results were used by many hospitals, resulting in creative and innovative changes. The initial proposal for the Magnet Hospital Recognition Program was approved by the board of directors of the American Nurses Association (ANA) in December 1990. The name was changed in 1996 to the Magnet Nursing Services Recognition Program for Excellence in Nursing Services. This change reflects the emphasis on providing national recognition for nursing service systems that attract and retain professional nurses and thus provide quality care. In 1998, the program was expanded to include a component that recognizes nursing excellence in long term care facilities. The magnet program is administered by the American Nurses Credentialing Center's (ANCC) Commission on the Magnet Recognition Program (*Nursing World* 2002b).

The overall goal of the magnet program is to identify excellence in the provision of nursing services and to recognize those institutions that act as a magnet by creating a work environment that recognizes and rewards professional nursing. Organizations interested in magnet recognition must first document their adherence to the ANA's Scope and Standards for Nursing Administrators. This lengthy document is reviewed by three ANCC appraisers; the appraisers determine if the organization meets the criteria to move to the next phase of the application process, the appraisal visit. The appraisal visit involves a site visit by two appraisers. As part of the process, ANCC seeks feedback from staff, clients, families, and the public. The program assesses excellence in several areas, including the following (*Nursing World* 2002b):

- management philosophy and practices of nursing services
- adherence to standards for improving the quality of patient care
- leadership of the chief nurse executive in supporting professional practice and continued competence of nursing staff
- attention to the cultural and ethnic diversity of patients and their significant others, as well as the care providers in the system

Magnet status recognition indicates excellence in nursing services, development of a professional milieu, and growth and development of nursing staff. Magnet recognition is valid for four years, after which time the recipient must reapply. Recognition of excellence may be publicized by the recipient and used in its marketing strategies directed toward both consumers and nurses. This may enhance recognition and reputation within the community and improve recruitment and retention of qualified professional nurses. Because the recognition award indicates excellence in nursing services, the recipient is a model for other nursing service systems (*Nursing World* 2002b).

At the time of publication, 55 facilities were recognized by ANCC as magnet facilities. Those facilities are listed in Table 12.1. Today, magnet-recognized facilities attract nurses by creating a positive work environment for nursing. Nurses are viewed as important contributors to patient care and the healthcare environment. RNs have autonomy in their practice and use their expertise and influence by participating in professional practice committees and interdisciplinary work groups. Not surprisingly, average nurse retention at magnet-designated facilities is twice as long as it is at nonmagnet institutions (Trossman 2002). Nurses in ANCC magnet hospitals reported higher levels of job satisfaction and lower burnout rates than in the hospitals identified in the original magnet hospital study (McClure et al. 1983). In addition, 89 percent of the nurses in ANCC magnet hospitals reported excellent or good quality of patient care compared to 75 percent of nurses in the original magnet study and 10 percent of nurses nationwide (Trossman 2002). In addition, studies suggest that patients in magnet facilities have better patient outcomes than those in other facilities (Trossman 2002).

CASE STUDY

University of Washington Medical Center (UWMC) in Seattle was one of the hospitals included in the original 1982–83 study by McClure and colleagues, and it was the first facility to earn ANCC magnet recognition. Staff nurses of all ages and levels of experience indicate a great deal of satisfaction in their work environment. An experienced staff nurse who graduated in 1957 stated, "Everyone wants to be here and is interested in improving patient care … It's also an affirming place to be. Nursing is respected by all departments." On the other end of the spectrum, a staff nurse with one and one-half years experience stated, "UWMC has a great atmosphere for learning. Every day I see something new, and the staff is great and very supportive of each other. I never feel alone … Everybody

Table 12.1: Healthcare Organizations with Magnet-designated Nursing Services

Arsitocrat Berea Skilled Nursing and Rehabilitation Facility
Berea, OH

Aurora Health Care: Hartford Memorial Hospital, St. Luke's Medical Center, St. Luke's South Shore, Sinai Samaritan Medical Center, and West Allis Memorial Hospital
Milwaukee, WI

Avera McKennan Hospital and University Health Center
Sioux Falls, SC

Baptist Hospital of Miami
Miami, FL

Bayfront Medical Center
St. Petersburg, FL

Capital Health System
Trenton, NJ

Catawba Valley Medical Center
Hickory, NC

Cedars-Sinai Medical Center
Los Angeles, CA

Children's Memorial Medical Center
Chicago, IL

East Jefferson General Hospital
Metairie, LA

Englewood Hospital and Medical Center
Englewood, NJ

Fox Chase Cancer Center
Philadelphia, PA

Hackensack University Medical Center
Hackensack, NJ

High Point Regional Health System
High Point, NC

Humility of Mary Health Partners
Youngstown, OH

Inova Fairfax Hospital
Falls Church, VA

James A. Haley Veterans' Hospital
Tampa, FL

Jersey Shore Medical Center
Neptune, FL

Jewish Hospital
Louisville, KY

Kimball Medical Center
Lakewood, NJ

Long Island Jewish Medical Center
New Hyde Park, NY

Mayo-Rochester Hospitals
Rochester, MN

Medical Center of Ocean County
Brick, NJ

The Methodist Hospital
Houston, TX

Middlesex Hospital
Middletown, CT

The Miriam Hospital
Providence, RI

Morristown Memorial Hospital
Morristown, NY

(continued)

Table 12.1 *(contined)*

Mount Sinai Medical Center
Miami Beach, FL

North Carolina Baptist Hospital
of Wake Forest University
Baptist Medical Center
Winston-Salem, NC

North Shore University Hospital
Manhasset, NY

Pennine Acute Services NHS
Trust: Rochdale Infirmary and
Birch Hill Hospital
Rochdale, Lancashire, England

Poudre Valley Health System –
Poudre Valley Hospital
Fort Collins, CO

Providence St. Vincent Medical
Center
Portland, OR

Riverview Medical Center
Red Bank, NJ

Robert Wood Johnson
University Hospital
New Brunswick, NJ

Rush–Presbyterian–St. Luke's
Medical Center
Chicago, IL

St. Francis Medical Center
Trenton, NJ

St. Joseph's/Candler
Savannah, GA

Saint Joseph's Hospital of Atlanta
Atlanta, GA

St. Joseph's Regional Medical
Center
Paterson, NJ

St. Luke's Episcopal Hospital
Houston, TX

St. Luke's Regional Medical Center
Boise, ID

St. Marys Hospital Medical Center
Madison, WI

St. Peter's University Hospital
New Brunswick, NJ

Southwestern Vermont Medical
Center
Bennington, VT

The University of Alabama
Hospital
Birmingham, AL

University of California, Davis,
Medical Center
Sacramento, CA

University of Colorado Hospital
Denver, CO

University of Kentucky Hospital
Lexington, KY

The University of Texas M.D.
Anderson Cancer Center
Houston, TX

University of Washington Medical
Center
Seattle, WA

West Boca Medical Center
Boca Raton, FL

Source: Nursing World (2002a).

working here—whether a nurse, an x-ray technician, or a dietitian—has a strong commitment to what they do and that helps make nursing easier" (Trossman 2002).

How did this happen? Not by sign-on bonuses and other short-term recruitment strategies. Instead, the UWMC leadership believes in building a culture that fosters and promotes nursing excellence. The director of patient care services explained, "We work very hard to have an environment that's an excellent place for nurses to practice." The chief nursing officer stated, "We are proud of our nursing magnet status. We have devoted significant resources to achieve and maintain this status because we know that nursing professionalism translates into the best patient care possible. It also enhances job satisfaction among our nurses and other staff who work here" (Trossman 2002).

Nurses are treated with respect and as legitimate members of the healthcare team. Nurse executives are on par with other hospital executives. Nurses are proud of their workplace and are secure and confident in their roles. UWMC has a long-term commitment to primary nursing, allowing for continuity of individualized care. Nurses make decisions about patient care without interference. They focus on improving patient care and serve on important interdisciplinary committees, such as a work group creating new sedation protocols for adult patients on mechanical ventilation. They develop nurse recruitment and retention strategies and determine hospital staffing needs four times a day. For new nurses, UWMC offers a year-long program that includes a three-month guided orientation, a new graduate symposium to build critical thinking and emergency management skills, and a peer support group (Trossman 2002).

UWMC is not immune to the impact of the nursing shortage. Many of its nurses are nearing retirement, and fewer new graduates are available to replace them. However, having characteristics in place that support magnet recognition allows UWMC to retain high-caliber nurses (Trossman 2002).

SUMMARY

The Magnet Nursing Services Recognition Program for Excellence in Nursing Services recognizes excellence in nursing services in healthcare organizations. Growing out of a 1983 descriptive study, the program emphasizes that a high-quality environment is vital to retaining high-caliber nurses. The magnet program addresses the work environment, nursing shortage, and quality of patient care (Foley 2002).

Building on previous chapters, the next chapter describes recommendations of key nursing groups and legislative issues related to nursing.

REFERENCES

Foley, M.E. 2002. "President's Perspective: It's a Small World." *The American Nurse*, p 4.

McClure, M.L., Poulin, M.A., Sovie, M.D., and Wandelt, M.A. for the American Academy of Nursing Task Force on Nursing Practice in Hospitals. 1983. *Magnet Hospitals. Attraction and Retention of Professional Nurses*. Kansas City, MO: American Nurses Association.

Nursing World. 2002a. "Magnet Facilities." [Online article; retrieved Sept. 24, 2002.] Washington, DC: American Nurses Association. http://www.nursingworld.org/ancc/magnet/magnet2.htm.

———. 2002b. "Magnet Nursing Services Recognition Program." [Online article; retrieved May 2, 2002.] Washington, DC: American Nurses Association. http://www.nursingworld.org/ancc/magnet.htm.

Trossman, S. 2002. "Nursing Magnets: Attracting Talent and Making It Stick." *American Journal of Nursing* 102 (2): 87, 89.

CHAPTER 13

Policy, Legislative, and Regulatory Issues

INTRODUCTION

A number of groups have identified policy, legislative, and regulatory issues related to nursing. The Tri-Council, made up of four powerful nursing groups, has issued recommendations related to several issues in nursing. The American Nurses Association, focusing on working conditions, has developed and is distributing a nursing bill of rights. Although nursing licensure is granted by individual states and has sometimes been viewed as a local issue, the federal government is addressing the areas of foreign nurses, nursing education, healthcare provider recruitment, and nurse retention. In addition, several states have addressed work life quality as it relates to mandatory overtime.

TRI-COUNCIL FOR NURSING POLICY STATEMENT

The Tri-Council is an alliance of the American Association of Colleges of Nursing (AACN), the American Nurses Association (ANA), the American Organization of Nurse Executives (AONE), and the

National League for Nursing (NLN). Each organization has a unique mission and functions autonomously. However, the four organizations are united by common values and meet regularly for dialog and consensus building in the areas of nursing work environment, healthcare legislation and policy, quality of healthcare, nursing education, practice and research, and leadership across all segments of the healthcare delivery system. The following sections of this chapter discuss the recommendations of the Tri-Council Policy Statement (2001).

The Tri-Council identifies a need to encourage the development and deployment of nursing personnel with skills appropriate to the healthcare system. Furthermore, it indicates that the public, policymakers, and the nursing profession must engage in ongoing, long-term workforce planning. Nursing recruitment and retention strategies are costly and must be implemented with some assurance that these efforts will be accompanied by specific strategies to overcome workforce issues that discourage long-term commitment to a career in nursing. The Tri-Council has made recommendations specific to education; the work environment; legislation and regulation; and technology, research, and data collection.

Education

The Tri-Council recommends a variety of education-based initiatives. It encourages the development of career progression initiatives, which include identifying the range of options available beyond entry-level positions, such as faculty, researcher, and administrator, and developing programs that will move nurses through graduate studies more rapidly. It also encourages a compensation system within the healthcare community based on an understanding of the educational preparation required for different nursing roles. The Tri-Council recommends that employers be supported in their efforts to create and sustain staff development programs and lifelong learning for continued nurse competence. Last, the Tri-Council encourages efforts to recruit younger and more diverse populations of nursing students by reaching out to youth through counselors, youth organizations, and schools.

The Work Environment

The Tri-Council recommends many initiatives related to the work environment. It suggests the implementation of specific strategies to retain experienced nurses in direct patient care. Such strategies might include greater flexibility in the workplace structure and scheduling, rewarding experienced nurses for serving as mentors and preceptors, and implementing appropriate salary and benefit programs. The Tri-Council recommends the creation of a partnership environment that advances nursing practice. This environment would include appropriate management structures, adequate nurse staffing, and nurse autonomy. The Tri-Council also addresses the needs of the aging nurse workforce, suggesting that work be redesigned so that older nurses can remain in direct care roles.

Legislation and Regulation

The Tri-Council makes two recommendations related to legislation and regulation. First, it recommends increased capacity and resources for education of the nursing workforce through increased nursing education funding under Title VIII of the Public Health Service Act and other publicly funded initiatives. Second, it advocates better identification of registered nursing services within Medicare, Medicaid, and other reimbursement systems.

Technology, Research, and Data Collection

The Tri-Council makes three recommendations in the area of technology, research, and data collection. First, it recommends that the use of technological advances to enhance the capacity of a reduced nursing workforce be investigated. Next, it encourages the federal Health Resources and Services Administration (HRSA) Bureau of Health Professions' Division of Nursing and other public or private organizations to develop models of health workforce planning that consider both the need and the demand for nursing services workforce planning. Last, it recommends the collection of consistent data at the local, state, and national levels to enable appropriate workforce planning for registered nurses.

AMERICAN NURSES ASSOCIATION

Since 1896, ANA has worked to shape the scope of nursing practice, the education for nursing practice, and the continuing competency for nursing practice (*Nursing World* 2002). As articulated by ANA, registered nurses promote and restore health, prevent illness, and protect people entrusted to their care. They help alleviate the suffering of individuals, families, groups, and communities. Nurses provide services that maintain respect for human dignity and embrace the uniqueness of each patient (ANA 2001). To maximize the contributions made by nurses, the dignity and autonomy of nurses in the workforce must be protected.

ANA has long served as an advocate for improvements in nurses' working conditions. In its efforts to aid nurses in improving their workplace and ensuring their ability to provide safe, quality patient care, ANA has developed the Bill of Rights for Registered Nurses. The impetus came at the Summit on Nursing Staffing meeting in May 2001, when more than 200 nurses identified the need for a document that would outline what nurses deserve and need to provide high-quality patient care in a safe environment. The Bill of Rights for Registered Nurses states that nurses have the right to a safe work environment, to practice in a manner that ensures the provision of safe care through adherence to professional standards and

Table 13.1: ANA's Bill of Rights for Registered Nurses

Nurses have the right to:
- practice in a manner that fulfills their obligations to society and to those who receive nursing care
- practice in environments that allow them to act in accordance with professional standards and legally authorized scopes of practice
- work in an environment that supports and facilitates ethical practice, in accordance with the Code of Ethics for Nurses with Interpretive Statements
- freely and openly advocate for themselves and their patients, without fear of retribution
- fair compensation for their work, consistent with their knowledge, experience, and professional responsibilities
- work in an environment that is safe for themselves and for their patients
- negotiate the conditions of their employment, either as individuals or collectively, in all practice settings

Adopted by the ANA Board of Directors, June 26, 2001.

Source: Reprinted with permission from the American Nurses Association; published by ANA, copyright 2001.

ethical practice, and to advocate on behalf of themselves and their patients (Wiseman 2001). The seven rights of nurses are summarized in Table 13.1.

The bill of rights will provide nurses in practice with a template with which to evaluate their current workplace. It will also help nursing students understand what to expect in the workplace. Adherence to the bill of rights will help institutions hire and retain qualified nurses. Nurses should work with their organization's recruitment and retention committee as well as the human resources department to ensure that provisions of the bill of rights are incorporated into appropriate policies and procedures (Wiseman 2001).

LEGISLATION FOR THE NURSING SHORTAGE

Federal legislation addressing the nursing shortage has been passed in the areas of the hiring of foreign nurses, funding for nursing education, and recruitment and retention in the health professions.

Foreign Nurses

In response to early concerns about nursing shortages in certain areas of the United States, the Nursing Relief for Disadvantaged Areas Act of 1999 was signed into law on November 12, 1999. The law allows qualified nurses from other countries to work in medically underserved areas in the United States, provided their employment does not negatively affect the wages and working conditions of American nurses. In addition, the law requires employers who hire foreign nurses to demonstrate that they are making efforts to reduce workforce shortages in the medically underserved areas in which they operate (Fitzgerald 2001).

Funding for Nursing Education

Early in his tenure, Department of Health and Human Services (HHS) Secretary Tommy G. Thompson identified the nursing shortage as a critical national priority. In September 2001, Secretary Thompson announced a new series of grants and contracts totaling more than $27.4 million to increase the number of qualified nurses and the quality of nursing services across the United States (U.S. HHS 2002).

The Nursing Education Loan Repayment Program (NELRP) is managed by the Bureau of Health Professions' Division of Nursing on behalf of HRSA, which is an agency of HHS. NELRP was appropriated $10.2 million for fiscal year 2002, reflecting an increase of approximately $8 million over the previous two years. This loan repayment program is designed to assist in recruitment and retention of registered nurses dedicated to providing healthcare to underserved populations. All NELRP participants enter into a contract agreeing to provide full-time employment in an approved eligible healthcare facility for two or three years. In return, NELRP will pay 60 percent of the participant's total qualifying loan balance for a two-year commitment or 85 percent of the participant's total qualifying loan balance for a three-year commitment (NIH 2002). Designation of areas having a shortage of RNs is made by the federal government based on the ratio of full-time-equivalent RNs to average daily census (ADC). Counties with an aggregate RN-to-ADC ratio in the lowest quartile of U.S. hospitals are designated as nurse shortage counties. This methodology could be improved by considering racial/ethnic composition and health insurance status, not just the RN-to-ADC ratio, when designating nurse shortage counties (Seago et al. 2001).

In an effort to address the nation's growing need for nursing professionals, President George W. Bush's fiscal year 2003 budget proposes a total of $15 million, nearly a 50 percent increase above 2001 funding, to expand the NELRP. The program repays a substantial portion of the education loans of nurses who agree to work for two years in designated public or nonprofit health facilities. A funding preference is given to nurses who have the greatest financial need and who agree to serve in health facilities located in geographic areas with the greatest shortage of nurses. The increase will support 800 new loan repayment agreements (U.S. HHS 2002).

Recruitment and Retention in the Health Professions

In February 2002, HHS Secretary Thompson and Department of Education Secretary Rod Paige launched a campaign to encourage school children to consider careers in nursing and the health professions. The education campaign, "Kids into Health Careers," makes information available on more than 270 health careers to students, parents, teachers, and organizations. For example, the kit includes content on the professions of nurse, physical therapist, x-ray technician, sports therapist, and emergency medical technician. The kit also includes information on the level of education preparation needed, salary outlook, and resources for obtaining financial assistance to pursue an education in the profession. Organizations that receive health professions grants through HRSA will be required to reach out to schools in their local communities to get more children involved in the health professions (U.S. HHS 2002).

The magnet program received national recognition when Senators Hillary Rodham Clinton (D-NY) and Gordon Smith (R-OR) introduced the Nurse Retention and Quality of Care Act. This federal measure, designed to remedy the nursing shortage, would provide grants to healthcare organizations to develop and implement model practices that the American Nurses Credentialing Center (ANCC) has identified as making the workplace more attractive (Trossman 2002).

WORK LIFE QUALITY LEGISLATION

In 2001, Maine and Oregon passed legislation prohibiting mandatory overtime for nurses. In Maine, the law indicates that no nurse may be disciplined for refusing to work more that 12 consecutive hours except in unforeseen circumstances in which overtime is required as a last resort to ensure patient safety. Nurses required to work in such situations will be given at least ten hours off before being required to work again.

Oregon's Safe Nursing Care Act limits mandatory overtime to two hours, enough time for the hospital to seek a replacement RN. Mandatory overtime cannot exceed 16 hours in a 24-hour period, although exceptions may be allowed during critical staffing shortages. The Oregon law also requires hospitals to develop and implement nursing staff plans. Hospitals must develop and use reliable classification systems, which will become the basis for RN staffing.

According to the law, the system should be based on individual patients' needs and intensity of the nursing care required. Clinical nursing staff members at each facility are to be part of the development, implementation, and ongoing evaluation process. To ensure compliance, the Oregon Health Division will audit at least 10 percent of hospitals each year. The health division is authorized to impose financial penalties when hospitals violate standards in the law. In addition, nurses are required to advise managers of their concerns about potential risks to patients and are protected when they report unsafe care or illegal activities internally. Last, nurses who believe they have suffered retaliation by their employers for protected activities may sue in court. The remedies include punitive damages (Farella 2001).

In March 2002, the state of Washington passed legislation prohibiting healthcare facilities from requiring registered nurses and licensed practical nurses to work more than 12 hours in a 24-hour period or 80 hours in a 14-day period, except in an emergency or when reasonable efforts to find volunteers or temporary staff to work have failed. On-call hours are excluded from the definition of overtime, and hospitals have the authority to require nurses to complete a procedure (*AHA News* 2002a). New Jersey (*AHA News* 2002b) and Minnesota (*AHA News* 2002c) have also passed legislation prohibiting mandatory overtime.

SUMMARY

This chapter has described recommendations of key nursing groups, including the Tri-Council recommendations and ANA's Bill of Rights for Registered Nurses. In addition, legislation related to foreign nurses, nursing education, recruitment, retention, and work life quality have been presented.

The book concludes with an afterword discussing a view of the future for nursing.

REFERENCES

AHA News. 2002a. "Washington Passes Bill Limiting Nurse Overtime to Emergencies." [Online article; retrieved Sept. 25, 2002.] Chicago: AHA. www.ahanews.com.

———. 2002b. "New Jersey Governor Signs Mandatory Overtime Prohibition." [Online article; retrieved Sept. 25, 2002.] Chicago: AHA. www.ahanews.com.

———. 2002c. "Minnesota Passes Bill Limiting Mandatory Overtime for Nurses." [Online article; retrieved Sept. 25, 2002.] Chicago: AHA. www .ahanews.com.

American Nurses Association (ANA). 2001. *The American Nurses Association's Bill of Rights for Registered Nurses.* Washington DC: ANA.

Farella, C. 2001. "Two States Pass Anti-OT Laws." *Nursing Spectrum* 14 (14IL): 5.

Fitzgerald, P.G. 2001. U.S. Senator, R-Illinois. Personal communication via e-mail, November 19.

National Institutes of Health (NIH). 2002. "Nursing Education Loan Repayment Program." [Online article; retrieved Sept. 25, 2002.] Washington, DC: NIH. http://bhpr.hrsa.gov/nursing/loanrepay.htm.

Nursing World. 2002. "Nursing's Agenda for the Future." [Online article; retrieved May 28, 2002.] Washington, DC: ANA. http://www.nursingworld.org/naf.

Seago, J.A., Ash, M., Spetz, J., Coffman, J., and Grumbach, K. 2001. "Hospital Registered Nurse Shortages: Environmental, Patient, and Institutional Predictors." *Health Services Research* 36 (5): 831–52.

Tri-Council. 2001. "Strategies to Reverse the New Nursing Shortage." Tri-Council Policy Statement. [Online article; retrieved Sept. 25, 2002.] Washington, DC: American Association of Colleges of Nursing. www.aacn.nche.edu/publications /positions/tricshortage.htm.

Trossman, S. 2002. "Nursing Magnets: Attracting Talent and Making it Stick." *American Journal of Nursing* 102 (2): 87, 89.

U.S. Department of Health and Human Services (HHS). 2002. [Online article; retrieved Feb. 2002.] Washington, DC: HHS. www.hhs.gov/news.

Wiseman, R. 2001. "The ANA Develops Bill of Rights for Registered Nurses." *American Journal of Nursing* 101 (11): 55, 57.

Afterword

In April 2002, a group of more than 60 nursing organizations released a strategic plan for addressing the nation's growing nurse shortage. The plan, entitled "Nursing's Agenda for the Future," targets ten areas for action (*Nursing World* 2002):

1. leadership and planning
2. delivery systems
3. legislation/regulation/policy
4. professional/nursing culture
5. recruitment/retention
6. economic value
7. work environment
8. public relations/communication
9. education
10. diversity

This plan may provide an additional road map for improving the climate of nursing.

Policies to address persistent shortages need to focus on distribution issues. RN workforce policy needs to place a greater emphasis on distribution relative to overall supply. Distribution policies include not only financial assistance programs but also programs that provide RNs with educational experiences in medically underserved communities and policies that seek to recruit into the profession individuals predisposed to practice in such communities (Seago et al. 2001). In particular, more attention should be given to recruitment of minorities and men into the nursing profession.

Nursing is, and always has been, a noble profession with a very positive public perception. Somewhere along the way, nursing lost faith in itself because of a combination of factors.

- In the eyes of the RN, nursing went from a profession to a job, because of dissatisfaction related to staffing, management, recognition and not having a voice in decision making.
- Nursing lost its luster as an attractive career option because of its own internal image problems and myriad alternative career options.
- Nurses themselves were aging and more interested in a way out for themselves, not a way in for the next generation. Role models were few and far between.
- Nurses allowed themselves to be the victim instead of the hero of the healthcare delivery system.
- Nursing leadership and academia remained divided on the future of nursing and the future of the nurse.

Can nursing reinvent itself? Can nursing be the healthcare profession of choice? Can nursing restore the pride inherent in being an RN? Can nursing become the "make a difference" profession in the evolving healthcare industry?

The answer is a resounding *yes*. Nursing is in the best position to be the "make a difference" profession. The healthcare industry is in a state of evolution or, perhaps, revolution. Customers are demanding more—more satisfaction with the healthcare experience, more information and disclosure, more guarantees of patient safety, and an expectation of positive outcomes after an encounter with any aspect of the healthcare delivery system.

Nurses are in the best position to meet these customer expectations. They have the education and expertise to greatly affect patient satisfaction. Emerging mandatory requirements in the patient safety arena will enhance both the role and the importance of nursing because of the documented impact that nurses and nurse staffing have on patient outcomes.

Fiscal concerns will continue to be a critical issue because of declining reimbursement and escalating operating costs. An economic case can be made for the role of the nurse in positively affecting the organization's bottom line.

Why do nurses have such a great impact on quality and cost?

- Nurses prevent complications, especially in the arena of nosocomial infections, urinary tract infections, pneumonia, thrombosis, and pulmonary compromise and decubiti.
- Nurses provide around-the-clock surveillance and proactively assess and monitor patient care, thus affecting directly patient care outcomes and length of stay.
- Nurses are the safety check between the physician and pharmacy; a higher nursing skill mix reduces medication errors.
- Nurses reduce liability and risk, which are both costly to institutions.

"Good catches," catching problems before they have an impact, are understudied in the literature; here, again, RNs affect both quality and cost. Good catches can prevent medication errors, injuries, wrong-side surgery, and other adverse events before they happen.

The future for nursing is bright. Few professions offer lifelong career opportunities that are flexible, challenging, recession-proof, and personally fulfilling.

FUTURE THINKING

A look into the crystal ball on nursing's furture shows both challenge and opportunity. The challenges are very real—the shortage of RNs is currently the most significant one. Yet opportunity lies in the national awareness and new funding that are occurring. New sources of funding are in process at the national and state levels and through philanthropy. Recently, Congress passed the Nurse Reinvestment Act, which will cost more than $30 million from 2003 to 2007 (U.S. Senate bill S.706, 2002). Major corporations are also getting involved.

Students and second-career professionals will consider nursing as a career option because of job and salary stability, demand, and flexibility to meet lifestyle needs.

Another challenge is escalating demand. The opportunity is in the advances in technology, which will enable nurses to spend less time on paperwork and more time on patient care. Alternative care models that focus on optimal utilization of RN skills and expertise represent another opportunity.

An aging workforce is a challenge and an opportunity. Physically demanding jobs are a challenge, yet the expertise and knowledge of the tenured RN can be harnessed in many ways—as clinical expert, mentor, preceptor, educator, senior clinician in virtual intensive care units, informatics expert, and clinical researcher.

Patient safety standards are a challenge for the healthcare industry, but a significant opportunity for nursing. Nurses have the expertise and availability to ensure patient safety, both proactively and via ongoing assessment.

The old adage, "there is safety in numbers" is true where patients are concerned. An August 2002 report of the Joint Commission on Accreditation of Healthcare Organizations, which analyzed sentinel events such as patient death or injury, identified low RN staffing levels as the cause in 24 percent of 1,609 cases (Joint Commission 2002). Hospitals with low RN turnover (under 12 percent) had lower adjusted scores on both patient mortality and length of stay. This is a compelling business case for retaining nurses and ensuring that adequate fiscal and human resources are available.

Net generation employees want to be in a "make a difference" profession; thus, it is critical to market nursing and the role of the nurse in patient safety with that in mind.

Magnet recognition for nursing is a challenge, in the rigor that is required both to apply and meet standards, and an opportunity, in the recognition it provides for nursing. Most nursing organizations will want to receive magnet recognition status because of its impact on recruitment and retention.

A last significant challenge is the working environment for nurses, yet, opportunities abound for a transformation within this arena. Technology as an enabler for nursing staff will transform documentation requirements. Creative and flexible working hours are becoming more common and will continue. Managers responsible for nursing are increasingly being held accountable as chief retention officers, so they are well-advised to provide a good work environment for their nurses.

WHAT DOES THE FUTURE HOLD?

We make the following predictions to bring this book to a close:

1. Increased nursing school enrollments will begin to be seen in 2004, with significant growth in accelerated second-degree programs.
2. Magnet certification will become a standard for nurses seeking positions.
3. Salaries will escalate at double the pace of inflation.
4. Public awareness and demand for nurses will escalate available funding for education and research.
5. Nursing research and nursing-driven outcomes will become as prevalent as other health services research, with higher levels of

funding, and articles discussing these issues will be published far more frequently in prestigious journals.

6. More men, minorities, and second-career professionals will choose nursing as a career.

7. Technology advancements will decrease non-patient-care tasks for nurses. Point-of-care charting, physician order entry, and clinician decision support will enhance RN job satisfaction.

8. Far more focus will be placed on multigenerational workforce management and meeting the needs of each segment of the nursing population.

Nurses of today and those contemplating the profession are legitimately concerned about patient care, patient safety, professional opportunities, and personnel safety. By making real changes in the work environment, we can realize a renewed and sustainable nursing profession.

REFERENCES

Joint Commission on Accreditation of Healthcare Organizations. 2002. "Health Care at the Crossroads: Strategies for Addressing the Evolving Nursing Crisis." [Online report; retreived Sept. 27, 2002.] Oak Brook, IL: JCAHO. www.jcaho.org.

Nursing World. 2002. "Nursing's Agenda for the Future." [Online article; retrieved May 28, 2002.] Washington, DC: American Nurses Association. http://www .nursingworld.org/naf.

Seago, J.A., Ash, M., Spetz, J., Coffman, J., and Grumbach, K. 2001. "Hospital Registered Nurse Shortages: Environmental, Patient, and Institutional Predictors." *Health Services Research* 36 (5): 831–52.

U.S. Senate Bill S.706. 2002. http://thomas.loc.gov/cgi-bin/query.

About the Authors

JULIE W. SCHAFFNER, M.S.N., R.N., is the chief operating officer and chief nurse executive at Advocate Lutheran General Hospital in Park Ridge, Illinois, a 609-bed teaching, research, and tertiary-care hospital and Level I trauma center. Mrs. Schaffner is responsible for the day-to-day operations of the hospital's clinical, ancillary, support, and nursing functions. She has served on numerous task forces and boards, including the *Journal of Nursing Administration* Editorial Board, the Advocate Home Care Board of Directors, and Midwest Children's Brain Tumor Center Advisory Board. Mrs. Schaffner has held positions as a staff RN, head nurse, healthcare consultant, and patient care executive and is an accomplished author and speaker in the healthcare arena. She received her M.S. and B.S. degrees from the University of Virginia and was a 1989 Johnson & Johnson Wharton Fellow.

PATTI LUDWIG-BEYMER, PH.D., R.N., is the administrative director for nursing research and education at Edward Hospital & Health Services in Naperville, Illinois. Edward Hospital is a 250-plus bed, full-service medical center. Dr. Ludwig-Beymer has 29 years experience in nursing, and she previously held positions in education, research, and clinical excellence at Advocate Health Care in Oak Brook, Illinois. In addition, she has been a staff nurse and faculty member in a variety of settings. She is a certified transcultural nurse and speaks and writes extensively. Dr. Ludwig-Beymer received her diploma in nursing from Mercy Hospital School of Nursing in Pittsburgh, Pennsylvania; her B.S.N. and M.S.Ed. degrees from Duquesne University in Pittsburgh, Pennsylvania; and her Ph.D. in nursing from University of Utah in Salt Lake City.